SOULOLOGY

DIS-EASE AND THE SOUL

The Soul's Encyclopedia for Dis-ease

DEBORAH L. CHEMOTTI &
SHAWNA L. TALBOT

Note for Librarians: a cataloguing record for this book that includes Dewey Decimal Classification
and US Library of Congress numbers is available from the Library and Archives of Canada. The
complete cataloguing record can be obtained from their online database at:
www.collectionscanada.ca/amicus/index-e.html
ISBN 1-4120-6544-5
Printed in Victoria, BC, Canada

Printed on paper with minimum 30% recycled fibre.
Trafford's print shop runs on "green energy" from solar, wind and other environmentally-friendly power sources.

TRAFFORD

Offices in Canada, USA, Ireland and UK
This book was published *on-demand* in cooperation with Trafford Publishing. On-demand
publishing is a unique process and service of making a book available for retail sale to the public
taking advantage of on-demand manufacturing and Internet marketing. On-demand publishing
includes promotions, retail sales, manufacturing, order fulfilment, accounting and collecting
royalties on behalf of the author.

Book sales for North America and international:
Trafford Publishing, 6E–2333 Government St.,
Victoria, BC v8t 4p4 CANADA
phone 250 383 6864 (toll-free 1 888 232 4444)
fax 250 383 6804; email to orders@trafford.com
Book sales in Europe:
Trafford Publishing (uk) Ltd., Enterprise House, Wistaston Road Business Centre,
Wistaston Road, Crewe, Cheshire cw2 7rp UNITED KINGDOM
phone 01270 251 396 (local rate 0845 230 9601)
facsimile 01270 254 983; orders.uk@trafford.com
Order online at:
trafford.com/05-1455

10 9 8 7 6 5 4 3 2 1

TABLE OF CONTENTS

ACKNOWLEDGMENTS v
PREFACE vii
1. A PARADIGM SHIFT OF DIS-EASE 1
2. THE GENETIC FACTOR 4
3. THE SOUL FACTOR...7
4. THE MESSAGE OF LEARNING 10
5. THE CAUSE AND EFFECT OF DIS-EASE....................................16
6. POTENTIALITY vs. LIMITATIONS
   POSSIBILITIES vs. IMPOSSIBILITIES 22
7. SOUL'S ENCYCLOPEDIA OF DIS-EASESEFROM A – Z 25
   INDEX..122

ACKNOWLEDGMENTS

M UCH THANKS and gratitude is given to many for their support during this project:

*We thank God for the gift of life and the opportunity to learn and share these truths with the world.

*I Deborah Chemotti am thankful for all things and everything that I have experienced in this vastness of life. I hold close to my heart my daughter throughout this journey. She was my angel of strength. I learned many things from her as we shared many things that only can be held as memories within my heart. I bow to her for her deep dedication for these writings to get to the masses, against all odds – at all costs. I couldn't of asked God for my two children and grandchildren to be any other way, for he has given me such miracles. There are no words great enough to express how I feel.

*I Shawna Talbot am thankful for my mother's valor and dedication to continue to have the fortitude to teach me the ultimate life truths under the ultimate conditions. She committed to discovering these truths, teaching them to me and sharing them with the world. This has been her soul's dedication. There was minimal recognition and encouragement to not give up and continue on. Yet, she motivated her own self. She stuck through it no matter what for these truths. She stopped at nothing, stood for her truths and pursued her soul's purpose at all cost. Truly she has been a gift to this world. She is my hero, my teacher, my friend and my mother.

*We thank White Eagle and all my spiritual guides for their guidance to help lead us throughout this journey.

*My son and brother Dr. Derek Talbot D. C. whom was one of the greatest pillars of strength and faith throughout this journey. He never quit believing in us.

*Our deceased mother and grandmother Irene Chemotti whom was the one that stood behind us, no matter what, with her care and support. Had it not been for her to care for my grandson and son Ryan Falzon during the progression of these books I would not have been given the chance to learn what my mother was teaching me. She always knew that it was our destiny to bring these truths to the world and we would not give up for nothing. Well, we made it thanks to you! We love you always.

*My grandson and son Ryan Falzon for learning these truths, following and teaching them as well as continuing to remind us how important it was for these books to get to the world.

*Donald Constable for his financial support and encouragement.

*Donald Carns for his financial support, emotional support and encouragement to get there.

*Many thanks to Dr. Mark Schaaf D. O. for being there, caring and understanding.

*Also, many thanks to all others whose paths we have crossed along our journey.

God Bless All,
Deborah Chemotti &
Shawna Talbot

PREFACE

THE GIFT

My mother Deborah Chemotti is the founder of Soulology, the study of the soul. She is the president of the Soulology Foundation, aimed at personal soul growth: awakening each individual to the true healer within. She is also the minister of The Church of Soulology. I Shawna Talbot am her daughter, student, Co-Founder of Soulology and the Vice- president of the Soulology Foundation.

The core of her quest was to understand the nature of dis-ease: What is dis-ease? Why do we have dis-ease? How can we overcome dis-ease? and "How can we prevent dis-ease?" Presently in this book we have the what, why and how we can overcome and prevent dis-ease, including the soulological causes; the reason why we have the dis-eases we do and the **soul learnings** we need to learn to overcome the dis-eases within this book.

Understand, the reason we refer to disease as dis-ease is because one is truly experiencing dis-ease. What are we really saying is that we are experiencing discomfort, unsettlement etc. within many parts of ones being. This dis-ease first occurs deep within our feelings, thoughts and spirit before our physical body experiences it. We call it dis-ease, because we are actually encountering DIS-EASE, at many levels, we are not at **ease** – in balance and in harmony within.

Before I could acquire the philosophy of dis-ease and learn how to apply this knowledge to work through dis-ease, my mother had to teach me many other life truths first. This took years of dedication. She taught me every day, nearly all day long. The knowledge she has taught me *seems* to be beyond any logical explanation. There weren't many things that I could spiritually ask her about life that she couldn't tell me. She had an innate knowing of these life truths, and the ones she didn't know she ventured to discover.

She taught me many learnings, concepts, theories and philosophies about life, not only about dis-ease and the different healing modalities, but also about our soul, our existence, our life; why things happen like they do and how to understand the messages coming from our soul to lead and guide us through life; getting in touch with the God within us and all around us; the understanding of the consciousness, how it works and how to expand its depths; and countless more truths. All these teachings were aimed at leading me to the understanding of dis-ease: What, Why and How.

Writing the Soulology series of books has been an ongoing process for us for many years. When I wrote down any of these teachings, I gave them back to her to see if I had understood and explained them correctly and fully. If not, she would re-write it and explain it to me. Not only did she teach it to me, she had to write it and rewrite it until it was right. It was vitally important that the truths speak clearly without confusion or any *some how's*. There is no question that she was born to share with the world these life truths, - the biggest truth of all being the understanding of dis-ease, how to prevent it and overcome it.

I believe a big trigger for her pursuit to understand the nature of dis-ease was that my brother was very sick as a child for many years. She knew that there had to be another way to approach dis-ease. She ventured to understand why there was dis-ease in the first place. "Why" was her quest for all of life's understandings. She didn't stop figuring and searching until she got the understanding. The effort was enormous. I came to see how quickly the average person will give up on understanding, just saying *"oh well*, or *somehow"*. Not her. She always said that everything has a purpose and it is divine, so that must be the case with dis-ease as well.

Throughout the years she has studied and researched different sciences, religions, medicines and alternative methods, using life as her laboratory. In her studies to understand life she needed a basis from which to determine, examine, measure and understand all things. She chose light (color) for her measurement of energy in life. All of life consists of light/color/energy and follows all of the same basic universal laws. And so she used color – energy in its simplest form - as her basis for understanding things.

She began with balancing color/energy in the body by therapeutically practicing color therapy. From a dream of a color therapy light table, came the creation of the color light table, built by my deceased grandfather Robert Chemotti. From there it evolved. She studied and practiced other alternative medicines to see their contributions. Eventually, together we therapeutically practiced about twenty alternative therapies.

We had our success stories. Then there are those who healed, only to have them return with a recurrence of the same dis-ease. To my mother these therapies were still not the true answer she was looking for: why were they not a success all the time in every case? Something was missing and she was going to search until she found it! She searched deeper into our beings: our mind, heart and spirit, until she reached the soul. The source of why there was dis-ease, that's where the answer was. Dis-ease comes from within – the soul!

She learned our soul is the source of who we are, which can be identified within our DNA. Our DNA consists of many genes. These genes represent specific characteristics. These genes are our strengths and faults; life lessons we have learned and lessons we have yet to learn within our ancestry, which we refer to as our soul learnings. These genes are passed on to us, and in part form our character, who we are today. They become a life outlook for us to excel in our strengths and acquire our soul learnings. This is how we grow and continue to evolve. Our ancestors pass on our soul's learnings, what our soul has come here to learn in order for our soul to grow.

Once my mother understood that dis-ease came from the soul's difficulty in learning its life lessons, acquiring its soul learnings, I began channeling the thoughts, feelings and beliefs associated with each dis-ease, gave them to her and then she began to determine what the soul learnings were for each of the dis-eases. However, she got more than she bargained for. She thought her genetics, as she would say, "Were stronger than they were." What was not innate knowledge, meaning soul learnings already acquired in her genetics, or learnings she acquired in her individual lifetime thus far, then she had to experience them in order to understand them. That is, she had to experience certain dis-eases to a greater or lesser degree, contingent on her degree of learning of them, as well as what else she needed to understand to figure out their soul learnings.

She had to go through much dis-ease to gain this knowledge. These times were very scary, especially at first. I saw her go through excruciating pain and suffering, facing dis-eases minor and major, such as back injuries, holes in her stomach, heart attacks, cancer, etc. Some of these dis-eases took longer than others to work through in order to come to understand the soul learning. When she was able to get the learning and then apply it, the dis-ease would exit her body.

It is only through such knowledge that the dis-ease can truly exit the body. It used to astonish me to see that it really did work that way. Once she got the learning, bingo!, the dis-ease was gone. It was like a miracle. Eventually, I began to understand dis-ease and applied this knowledge. I indeed experienced the same miraculous process. Since then, many others have also applied this knowledge to work through their dis-eases.

Through this journey to understand dis-ease I came to learn that the true spiritual path was about selflessness and compassion, both of which she taught to me and reflected to me daily. The most important of all her teachings was compassion – "others"; as she would say. *Life is God's gift to us and what we do with it is our gift back to God.* In life, we have a chance to reflect and be thankful for all that we have been given, and then we get the opportunity to give to others in return for our thanks. We are the most thankful people on this earth for these **gifts** of truths that have been given to us to share with others.

By Shawna Talbot

1

—⊰⊱—

A PARADIGM SHIFT
OF DIS-EASE

Dis-ease is not meant to make us suffer, rather it is a reminder from our soul that we are growing, evolving and learning new ways to cope and adapt to our life and its environment. Within our realm of existence there is a positive and negative nature within all things. This principle includes dis-ease as well. The law of purpose tells us that everything happens for a reason. Even though experiences at times appear negative, everything is perfect in its progression. Dis-ease is not bad, and it just didn't accidentally happen; it is part of a divine plan. It is part of evolution, our progression forward. The positive nature of dis-ease is that it provokes many of our soul learnings. This is in fact why we acquire dis-ease. Every dis-ease represents a process of our growing. Dis-ease is a last attempt to make us deal with what our soul must learn in order to overcome the dis-ease and continue to grow. Dis-ease is an opportunity to enhance who we are as personal beings as well as a whole species.

Each situation and circumstance that we experience in our life is an opportunity for our soul's growth. Life experiences provide us with the opportunity to learn our soul learnings in order for our soul to grow and continue to evolve. We go through many different experiences, both positive and negative in nature, so that we can learn. Experiencing different situations in our life requires us to deal with certain *soul learnings*, which in actuality are the specific *life lessons* that we are here to learn. If we cannot learn these life lessons, they eventually emerge into dis-ease.

Every experience that we as individuals encounter throughout life has a message from our soul for our learning. By becoming consciously aware of this positive realization, we are able to see that life is trying to offer us understanding through these experiences. As we encounter these learnings, we can choose to either face them or ignore them. If we ignore the learning, it only harbors within us and, over time, eventually creates dis-ease in the physical body.

Every dis-ease has a soul learning behind it, its soulological cause, the reason why. To truly eliminate the dis-ease from one's body, one needs to deal with the soul learning. This learning will show itself again and again even through many generations until we face it, accept it, come to terms with it and apply it into our lives. The sooner we are able to deal with the soul learning, the sooner the dis-ease can exit the body.

The objective is to eventually learn to identify, accept and face our soul learning's at the subtle levels, through our life experiences, before they have to reach the physical body. Our feelings, thoughts and beliefs are in dis-ease before our physical body ever is. If we can catch the soul learning at these subtle levels, emotionally, mentally and spiritually coming to terms with the learning there, then we can learn to prevent dis-ease from reaching the physical body. In too many cases however, the soul learning has already escalated to the point that the dis-ease will emerge in the physical body for that learning.

Dis-ease in the physical body is the last stage for us to acquire our soul learnings in order for our souls to continue to evolve further. Once dis-ease reaches the physical body, the learning becomes much harder to learn. Remember, the dis-ease didn't get there overnight, so for the most part we won't be able to eliminate it overnight. The healing can take a short time or a lifetime. There is no miraculous cure that we can go looking for. We will not find it. Overall, we can only truly heal ourselves. Yes, the external has many *tools* to help us, but it is only through ourselves that we can truly heal ourselves. Once the dis-ease reaches the physical body, the only means for eliminating it is to come to terms with the soul learning, which is the true cause for the dis-ease. When we do this, the dis-ease can then exit the body. With understanding comes the *ease*.

Our purpose in writing this book is to aid in the healing process by bringing others *truths* about many understandings in life, including the process of dis-ease, how to overcome it and how to prevent it. These truths help one to understand how to prevent dis-ease before it reaches the physical body, as well as how to overcome it once it has reached the physical body.

Our intention is to try to help others to increase their level of awareness as to how they can heal themselves by understanding the purpose of dis-ease. The true healing process is only done through our self, from within. *We are all our own healers by divine plan.* No single being can heal another being. We can only truly heal ourselves. Other individuals may be key players in providing the guidance one needs to heal oneself, but the *self* and only the *self* can heal the *self*. It is not our objective to heal another, but rather to share with others what we have learned that has helped us, and many others.

In this book we offer many different tools that help us understand what our soul is trying to get us to learn, as well as the soul learnings for numerous dis-eases from A-Z. We can use the tools offered in this book to help us identify our soul learnings to understand them before it has to emerge into dis-ease at the physical body, as well as once it has reached the stage of dis-ease at the physical body. .

2

THE GENETIC FACTOR

WHEN WE look at the biological body for the meaning or the cause of dis-ease, we often say that it is genetic. Yet, we leave people in great mystery of genetic meaning simply that we acquired it from our ancestors for some unknown reason. Each gene that is passed on to us from our parents is not random at all, but rather divinely chosen to make up the unique individual that we are. They are precisely chosen for each individuals soul's specific soul learning. This is how we evolve. These genes are our character strengths and weaknesses; which are the immunities and learnings passed on to us from our parents and ancestors. Our genes determine the strengths and learnings each unique individual acquires in their life.

What dis-ease one is or is not likely to acquire is indeed based on ones genes. What each one of our ancestors did or did not learn gets passed down to the next generation as both strengths, which are our immunities, as well as weaknesses, which are soul learnings not yet acquired. Therefore, there are certain dis-eases that one would not be prone to acquire because one's ancestors have already learned the lesson associated with it. Through their learnings, it has already become a strength within the bloodline, and thus their descendants will have an immunity to the dis-ease. However, there are certain dis-eases that we are prone to or genetically set up for, known as our weaknesses, due to our lack of growth. If we do not acquire the learning our soul has set/lied out for us then dis-ease is most likely to emerge.

We come into life having certain strengths, as well as certain weaknesses, which are areas of learning that we need to obtain. If we do not learn this then dis-ease can emerge. Dis-ease can start at the instant of birth or occur somewhere along our journey of life. This is contingent on where our soul is at as far as obtaining our soul learnings. If one comes into life with a particular dis-ease, it is because right off the beginning there is immediate learning needed for continued soul growth.

As we travel through life, if we obtain the learnings needed for our soul, then the learning does not have to turn into dis-ease. If we can acquire our soul learning at the subtle levels, such as through dis-ease within our thoughts, feelings and beliefs we can then prevent the dis-ease from reaching the physical body. Dealing with dis-ease at the subtle levels saves a lot of experiences and suffering because we are now consciously working on the soulological cause, where our learning resides, instead of trying to just fix the symptoms in our physical body without knowing the reason why they are there.

Everyone will at some time face some type of dis-ease, as they face difficulty in learning what their soul has required of them. We all have our own individual soul learnings that will be challenging for us to overcome. At times when we are having a lot of trouble obtaining the understanding for our soul learning then we are potentially vulnerable to dis-ease. Throughout this process of obtaining our soul learnings at times **our bodies will become weakened, our hearts torn, our minds disassembled and our spirits shattered.** It is certainly not the easiest journey, but it is the most fulfilling and empowering journey that you will ever discover.

Upon entering life, we all have lessons to learn to further enhance our soul – that's the objective! The objective of life is to give us the chance to learn by presenting experiences for us to encounter so that we can obtain the life lessons needed. Our life is genetically set up for us to deal with these soul learnings. Our soul starts this preparation at conception. At that time we begin planning and setting our life up so that we will have the opportunity, a life style, that will prove promising for our soul to accomplish such a task. This is not necessarily "promising" in the terms that you may be thinking of, such as a life that is all positive and wonderfully joy-filled. Rather, we are given many opportunities that will best help us to learn what we must. Learning to look at the positive aspect in all experiences both positive and negative is where you'll find the answer – learning, not by getting caught up in only the negative aspect of the experience.

We need to realize as human beings that the life that we live today is NOT the big picture. Life is not about living for just the body and life's pleasures that we exist in today. Certainly, bodily pleasures are part of it, and frankly without the body we would not have the opportunity to learn and experience life. Yet, truly life is about living for the purpose and intention of the soul. If we are only looking at the smaller picture, it is very hard to comprehend how and why we experience the things that we do.

The life that we live today is only a fraction of the life of our soul. Our soul has had many lives before this one and will continue to have many lives after this one. Although it may seem like this statement makes this life sound so insignificant, such is not the case. Without the body that we are presently living in, we would not be able to hear the crackling of the leaves, smell a flower, see a sunset, feel the raindrops on our face or taste a homemade apple pie. Our body is very vital to our soul; the soul cannot obtain growth without it. The soul cannot experience without a body, and if the soul cannot experience, then it cannot have the opportunity to learn, and thus it cannot grow. It is very important that we take good care of our body and respect it. We need to be good to ourselves. The soul grows and advances in stages. In other words, all the experiences that we have gone through in all of our life, including our genetic ancestry, have been the building blocks to form who we are today. We all have had an easier time learning some things and a more difficult time learning other things. The experiences that we encounter are matched to our individual strengths and weakneses in a way that will best help us learn. Our soul has been through so many lives and so many experiences and that variety is what makes us the unique individuals that we are today. People enter a life that is uniquely prepared for their particular soul growth in his or her journey of life - learning.

3

THE SOUL FACTOR

EACH OF us is on a journey of life orchestrated by our soul. Captive within our souls are the blueprints of our map for life. These blueprints contain information about the journeys that our soul has traveled, our soul's current destination, and the plans for our soul's future destinations. These blueprints are encoded in each and every one of us, within our DNA. *Our genetic code is indeed our soul's code for learning.*

Our soul is a combination of both our mother and father's souls: their two souls have merged to create a new soul. Our father and mother's soul's consist of all they have learned in their lives, as well as all that their ancestors have learned, leading all the way back to the beginning of the original soul.

The other determining factor that contributes to our soul is all of the life experiences and learnings that we ourselves have personally encountered and acquired throughout our individual lives. All of this knowledge is stored within our soul imprinted in our DNA. This knowledge is the basis for who we are and what we need to now accomplish in our life in order for our soul to further grow and evolve.

To better understand this process, we will *briefly* touch on the meaning of reincarnation. *Reincarnation* plays its part in the pathway of life's divine plan through the process of procreation. As we procreate new life, we continue to pass down from generation to generation through the eons, all the things that our soul has learned, as well as the things that we still need to learn in order for our souls to continue to grow. This heritage consists of many lifetimes of experiences.

Depending on the different learning's for the vast individual beings that we are, it can take days, months, years, generations, even eons to acquire some of these soul learnings. How long this process takes depends on how much knowledge was passed down to us from our ancestors, as well as how much we have experienced and learned of a particular soul learning ourselves in our life time thus far. This factor will relate to the degree of learning and struggle we will go through in our life to acquire our soul learnings. For some of us it will be easier, while others could have to endure much more for the learning.

For example, within our previous ancestry if there has not been a lot of learning for a particular soul lesson, then we will have to go through a lot more experiences to gain the understanding of our soul learnings. On the other hand, if our ancestors have gained a lot of learning about a particular soul lesson, then obtaining this particular soul learning will be less challenging, and we may be able to complete it, therefore turning this learning into a strength.

Whether we have traveled different or similar paths to get where we are today, we have all become unique individuals with different strengths and weaknesses by traveling the roads designed by our unique soul for our individual soul learnings. The journey that we need to travel in our life becomes our life's purpose. Every living thing receives its purpose from its soul. Everything in life must have a purpose to fulfill or it could not exist. Without purpose there is nothing to strive for.

Our life is designed within the blueprints of our soul, mapped out within our DNA, to accomplish our life's purpose. The objective is to learn how to read our soul's map so that we can stay in close alignment with our life's purpose. Within each of us is an internal compass – our soul. Our soul guides us throughout our life; through our gut feelings, intuition, experiences, people, places and things, such as t. v. , radio, billboards, bumper stickers etc. There are many *signs* within us and around us that are continually coming from our soul to convey messages to help us navigate ourselves through life. By paying attention to these signs from our soul, within and without, we are able to align ourselves with our soul's intentions, therefore helping us to learn our life lessons.

The more clearly we align ourselves with obtaining our soul learnings, the fewer unpleasant experiences we will have to face. Each time we go through an experience to help us acquire our soul learning and we don't come to an understanding of it, the next experience gets a little bit harder, and then harder still, until our soul gets the soul learning that is needed. Dis-ease is one of the unpleasant processes that can arise if we do not acquire the particular soul learning that we need, this process is the main focus of this book: the soulological causes for our biological dis-eases. This book presents the context of the soul learning's for many dis-eases so that readers can begin to understand the soulological cause of their dis-eases to better be able to face and learn the lesson being presented to them by their soul. Until the understanding is learned the dis-ease cannot be eliminated from the being. The only way dis-ease can truly be eliminated from the being is through the understanding of it.

Dis-ease is one of life's many processes that we go through to try to learn our life lessons. Dis-ease emerges as a last resort to get our attention when we are having difficulty processing through our soul learnings in life. Every dis-ease is related to a soul learning. Dis-ease emerges through the adaptation of these soul learnings. By coming to understand and learn what our soul is trying to convey to us through the process of dis-ease, we can then address it, learn it and thereby overcome it.

Every experience we encounter is for the purpose of soul growth. There are no accidents or coincidences; rather, every experience, including dis-ease, has a message of learning in it for us. To understand our soul learnings we must learn to look to our life experiences and evaluate what they are trying to tell us. By understanding our soul learnings through our life experiences at the subtle levels: mentally, emotionally and spiritually we can then learn to prevent dis-ease from manifesting in the physical body. Through our life experiences, both by externally understanding our soul signs and by internally learning to listen to what our soul is conveying to us, we can live a healthy, happy and more harmonious lives.

4

THE MESSAGE
OF LEARNING

O<small>N A</small> daily basis, all opportunities for learning our souls lesson present themselves to us in our passing day to get our attention and invite us to gain some learning from them. Another way that we can capitalize on our learning is by watching others' experiences, and then reflect on them what learning is being conveyed to us. If we were a witness to the other person's experience, then the experience was offering us something to learn from it as well. Although it was another's experience, we didn't see it by accident, there was something for us to learn from it or we wouldn't of seen it. We are all put on this earth together to learn from one another. Everyone has something that they can teach. This is why we are all here together, to reflect to each other our learnings. Nothing is by accident. We need to remember that we were present for that experience for a reason, and the reason is that there is learning for us to get from it. Therefore, we should be asking ourselves, "What is this saying to me?""What is my soul trying to convey to me for my learning?"

Every experience that we encounter in life, whether it be big or small, is there for **us**; that is why we were there to see it, hear it, etc. Think about everything we see, hear, smell, taste and touch in one day alone. We take in a numerous amount of stimulus - information, both consciously and subconsciously. All of this has meaning to us. They are all messages trying to tell us something. Everything in life that we run

10

across has a message for us, either reflecting something to us that we are needing to learn and adapt into our character. Our job is to find out what the message is.

The experiences that we encounter in our everyday lives are like little reminders to better help us obtain our soul learnings. No one is going to always be there to help us through life, pointing out all of the do's and don'ts. This is our job, through which we learn by practice and experience. Life is full of these reminders that guide us about what to do and what not to do. Often we are just unaware of them. Life is like a game of clues. We set out with a purpose to capture learning, yet the details are unique for each of us.

For every experience that we go through, we do gain something from it. It is really a matter of *how much* of it we were able to learn each time. What we got out of one experience will now prepare us to take on another experience. Even again, we may not get all of it, maybe only some, so we will encounter yet another experience until the learning is completed. These new experiences presents us with the same type of learning from a different perspective. If it is still not learned in our lifetime then it is passed on to the next generation until it is learned.

When it comes to our learning, it is not going to be easy to learn. We are going to reject a lot of experiences that come into our lives because these weaknesses are such a strong part of our character that we don't truly know how to be any other way. Our objective now is to understand it, but this doesn't always come easy.

To acquire the soul learning, one must first face the learning at hand that is causing distress to one's being. Yet, we cannot face the learning unless we know what the learning is and understand it. Therefore, we need to bring the learning into consciousness. At first when we are trying to understand it, there is no clarity. To get to this point of clarity, where the learning is seen and understood, we will go through experiences that will bring to us more understanding. Once it is conscious then we are able to deal with it. First, we need to realize it. Then we must accept it and face it, in order to understand it, so that we can then deal with it and overcome it.

The dis-ease process is centered around surfacing the soul learning that is buried deep within us, to bring it to a point where it is clear, conscious. The learning presents itself in such a manner so as to surface clearly to our consciousness the different parts of our character that may be in question, for example, selfishness, insecurity, etc. It is presented to us in a way that we are actually showing ourselves constructive criticism and how to reconstruct our character. These experiences will encourage waves of distress because it is hard for us to deal with this uprooting of our character, being shown our faults and realizing that we must change. It can be very difficult to face and accept our soul learning, and therefore we may not be ready and willing to make the changes yet.

When learnings are first surfacing, we will notice unexplained feelings that arise. An emotional upheaval is taking place that is unburying suppressed feelings that never got answered or expressed; they were just left to dwell inside us. They never go away if they are not satisfied or understood; they just stay stored and wait for another opportunity to be expressed. They arise at times when we don't necessarily understand why. The reason they surface later, similar in some form, yet very different in others, is because they remind us of the experience that we went through when the feeling was suppressed in the first place. This is part of the process, re-experiencing similar circumstances to bring the feelings to the surface. These experiences rise in our life to help pull out these buried feelings so that we can try to satisfy them once and for all by understanding them, coming to terms with them, and overcoming them.

The reason we suppress these learnings in the first place, which eventually leads to dis-ease, is because we lack the understanding for them. We haven't yet acquired the necessary skills or understanding to gain this soul learning. If one cannot get the learning through these experiences, then this lack of learning continues on, eventually leading to dis-ease in the body. Then the dis-ease becomes the necessary type of experience needed to acquire the soul learning. Yet, how we can work through the dis-ease is by gaining this knowledge, the soul learning, and then the dis-ease can exit the body.

As soon as discomfort arises we need to take the time to pay attention to what we are experiencing from a situation. Any time we feel discomfort, we should try to look back at the experience and determine "What thoughts and feelings arose?""What brought about this distraught?""Why did this make us feel uncomfortable?"We need to look at what exactly we are having a hard time with. "What is my soul needing to learn here?"By taking time to look for our growth potential, we are then facing the situation, accepting it, and then we will be able to apply it into our life pattern, thus turning it into a strength. This is the objective for all of our soul learnings.

Many people ask, "How do you deal with your soul learning once you really know what it is?"First of all, understanding the soul learning is not as easy as, "Oh, I've realized a learning; okay now I'll just adapt my character accordingly and bring myself into balance. "This change takes a lot of patience, time, discipline, practice and commitment - daily. It's a lot tougher than you think. What it boils down to is this: it is hard to change.

The problem is that life is not predictable: it is about growth, which requires change. We as individuals often do not like change; it is uprooting. The reason we don't like change is because we automatically assume that if we agree to change, we are admitting that we were wrong or were not good enough. Really it is quite the opposite, change says that we are growing and learning. If we are not changing, then we are going nowhere. We need to learn to accept the idea of what change means to us. Change means growth, and this is what we are all really here for.

Experience is the key to our growth. This is why our lives are programmed so that we go through the experiences that lead us to the understanding needed for our soul learnings. It is necessary to take some time and evaluate our experiences. This evaluation is in fact a form of facing the soul learning. When evaluating the life experiences presented to us, we need to look for our areas of growth that are being presented to us in the experiences. In every experience, there is something that is trying to be conveyed to us for our learning. We must be *truthful* and *honest* with ourselves when evaluating these experiences. Looking at these situations objectively and be ready to make some changes in our self. Change is good, although so many of us fear it. We like to hang on to the familiar because it's secure. It may not be the best, but we know all the general rules; there is no risk involved. This is truly an unsuccessful way to live life.

When we are first presented with a lesson of learning, we experience emotional distress because we are unable to deal with it. Then mental disharmony comes along, because we can't place it. We cannot place it because we cannot relate to it, because we have little to no past experiences to refer to for understanding. After this reaction, we learn to live with this disharmony within, because we don't know how to deal with it, and thus it becomes a part of our character. Over a period of time the body begins to be programmed with this disharmony, which in fact creates the disease. Different types of learning's create different types of dis-eases. Unfortunately, it is only when the process gets to the point of dis-ease in the physical body that we begin to pay attention, because we feel biological discomfort and pain.

In common practice, we suppress the learning by taking medication or using alternative means to alleviate the symptoms and discomfort, so that we can go on our way and don't have to deal with the true cause. However, if we are consciously working on our learning and using external help such as medication or alternative means as a tool, these external aids can be very helpful. By working on the learning we stay conscious of it. By being conscious of our learning while using additional tools, we are not trying to avoid the learning and using the tools as a crutch, but rather using the tools to help us work through our soul learnings.

The only true way to eliminate dis-ease from the body is through understanding its cause. This is done by facing the soul learning. That is, no longer trying to suppress the discomfort the body feels by ignoring the learning. Our body is giving us warning signs from our soul. This is the way our body and soul communicate to us that something is not right. We need to not suppress the uncomfortable signs our body is feeling. We could save ourselves much discomfort by realizing the soul learning and agreeing to take on its calling, heading toward understanding this learning and turning this into a strength.

Once we have become consciously aware of our soul learning, then we need to accept it. By accepting it, it naturally begins to play a part in our life. Once it is conscious, we begin to portray ourselves in such a manner to accommodate our newfound understanding. As we begin to display this change in our character, the world external to ourselves will begin to change. Opportunities will be presented to us so that we can begin to make changes in our character. This happens when we put our understandings into application, by adapting ourselves in such a way to comply with our newfound learning. We take what we have learned from our weakness and turn that part of our character into a strength. The hardest part of this we have already accomplished, namely, surfacing it, facing it, accepting it and understanding the learning. Now we must work towards applying our new knowledge. This is a learning cycle, the turning of a weakness into a strength. At the end there is the gain – the soul learning, which is now a strength that has become a complete part of our character. At this point we no longer have to face this learning; it has been learned and will now be passed down through the generations as a strength.

We must realize that we are here to learn, and that every experience that we encounter throughout our lives occurs for a reason and has a particular purpose to serve. So many of us are going through life blind, hitting our heads up against the wall and not even knowing why.

We need to open up to the fact that we are here to learn, and the way we learn is by going through the many life experiences positive and negative in store for us. The sooner we realize this, and thus look at our life experiences as circumstances presented to us so that we can learn something from them, the sooner we can start to catch the message of learning that is being conveyed to us at the subtle levels, from a preventive point of view, instead of waiting until it reaches dis-ease at the physical level.

We can practice this method through every experience that we encounter, taking time to be honest and evaluating them, asking ourselves, "What is this experience that I am encountering trying to convey to me from my soul for my learning?" After taking time to train ourselves to do this with true honesty, then we will naturally reach a point where our lessons are no longer quite as traumatic, and they do not have to lead into dis-ease at the physical body.

Once we are able to realize the message of learning and accept it, then we are able to adapt this learning into our character; therefore, we won't have to encounter any greater experiences of tragedy or dis-ease in relation to that learning. This is how we can save ourselves a lot of grief.

5

THE CAUSE AND EFFECT OF DIS-EASE

I**F WE** want to win this battle of dis-ease, we must understand the cause behind the dis-ease, the soul learning. Not until we can understand the true cause, will we able to master the dis-ease. We can never be free from dis-ease until we can understand the purpose behind it – it's cause. By blaming the external, we will never find the true *cause*, the *why* for the dis-ease.

In our world we are on a great search to find the *cure* for dis-ease, yet we will never find the cure until we complete the search for the cause – the reason why, its purpose. Usually, the only time we spend trying to discern the cause for our dis-ease is when we have no magic medicine to take. Once we have the medicine, we don't care about the *cause* or about managing our lives in ways that will lead us to understand the nature of our illness – its purpose.

Medicines and alternative therapies are suppose to be used as tools to help us through our dis-ease process. Unfortunately, when we are working on our soul learning, sometimes these tools can end up becoming crutches. These tools are there to be used while we are consciously going through our soul learning. They are not to be used as crutches to avoid dealing with our soul learnings.

To cure is to eliminate or fix, and by no means can we fix any problem if we don't understand what is truly causing it. We will only forever be putting bandages

16

on leaking wounds. Even when we have what is deemed *the cure*, there is really no curing involved. Often we are just fixing it by altering it, taking it out, or so forth, so that it *appears* OK. It appears cured because we have removed the *seen*, but the *unseen* still remains in great agony.

Medicine has designed ways to artificially fix the body with surgery, yet they are not fixing the problem, but rather eliminating the symptoms. This would be a nice approach if the dis-ease were truly eliminated, yet this is not so. The seen is eliminated, so we naively think that the dis-ease is gone. Yes, the dis-ease may not be *seen* or felt in the physical body at the present time. Yet, the whole being is not free from the dis-ease, and it is sure to show itself again in another form, or maybe even the same form after a period of time. If not, it will be passed down to future generations, because the soul learning; the cause, was not learned.

For example, when people have cancer, the cancer may be cut out of the body, yet it is still continuing to create itself, not only in their minds and bodies, but throughout their lives as well. They live in the cancer around them, which is within them. We can cut the cancer out of the body, but we cannot cut it out of our life. The only true resolution is coming to terms with it by realizing the soul learning and accepting it in order to understand it and overcome it.

To take another example, if the brain is unable to produce a chemical balance to the body, then just because we artificially supply the body with the chemical that it is unable to produce on its own at this time, then we assume we have *cured* it – fixed the body. The body only appears fixed because the seen is in balance, yet the unseen still remains very ill. And for this there are consequences. If the unseen remains ill, we have stopped way too short of the real cause, and for this we will have to go through this process again, if not in our lifetime, then certainly in our future generations. In time, there is no doubt that the unseen will make itself seen again, until it is learned.

In searching deeper for the understanding of the cause for dis-ease other than the external, we are driven farther back into the inner workings of the being. Dis-ease has been linked to one's way of thinking and one's feelings in a way that it causes disharmony to the body. The way we think and feel clearly affects the body in numerous ways. Many studies have been done indicating how our thoughts and our feelings affect every cell within our body.

True, our thoughts affect our body and also involve our feelings, because our thoughts and feelings are both centered in the mind. Our feelings do not come from our heart. Our feelings are centered in a place within the brain. Both our thoughts and feelings come from our brain. Our brain sends out signals to the body of what it is thinking and feeling, and the body sends the messages back, to and fro. If, for example, we are feeling inadequate, then this signal of feeling inadequate is constantly being sent throughout the body. Overtime, this same negative signal being sent to the body will eventually create dis-ease within the body. When someone stays stuck in this state of feeling inadequate, then that message is being sent to every cell in the body over and over. The results will most likely end in dis-ease.

For example: When someone says an affirmation such as, "I feel adequate", the brain thinks that thought and thus that hormone gets released throughout the body. But because there is so much of the rest of the brain that is still continually sending out the message of "inadequacy" that they are thinking and feeling about themselves, reprogramming this little dose of worth or "adequate" is not going to work. The little bit of "I feel adequate" is not nearly making up for the rest of them that is thinking and feeling that "I don't feel adequate. "That is the way they truly feel and think about themselves based on their life experiences. Not until they address the soul learning, by coming to feel adequate within them self can the dis-ease in relation to inadequacy exit the body. The only way we learn to feel adequate is through life experiences that show us that we are indeed adequate.

Deep within we feel inadequate and we are sending that message throughout our body every day. And until we can come to see ourselves as adequate through our life experiences, our body is going to be affected by that message. We must go deeper and figure out why we are feeling inadequate: What has caused these feelings, few or many?When we understand this then we will be able to make further progress.

As we go through life, we see life through a personal perspective based on how we have come to view life and things in life. How we view life and the circumstances that we face in life is based on our personal experiences. Our perception of something creates a mindset (state of mind) based on how we felt at the time. Thus, our mindset is a state that is created and comes to run our being. The way we think and feel affects our whole body. Every cell within the body will become that mindset, whether the thoughts and feelings be joy or anger.

Although we can live in a state of joy forever and never have any problems, we cannot live in a state of anger without problems. If from our perspective we are viewing our life and the circumstances of our life with anger, then our whole body exists in this state of anger. Every cell within exists in anger. Think about it: How long can a cell exist in anger without becoming angry itself?Once it becomes angry the effect shows through in the body, often leading to dis-ease.

There are many different dis-eases that are created by many different types of thoughts and feelings - emotions. Different emotions produce certain states of mind that affect particular cells and parts of the body differently, thus leading to different types of dis-eases. The type of dis-ease one ends up with depends on what one is thinking and feeling due to one's own individual soul learnings in life. The cause for our dis-ease is not something in the external world; rather it is an internal process that is triggered by external means. Although the external is not the *cause* of dis-ease, it plays a big part in the *triggering* of dis-ease.

For example, researchers have linked death from lung cancer and smoking. Yet, what about the people who died of lung cancer but never smoked a day in their life, as well as those that did smoke, yet never had any lung problems. Here we see inconsistency in blaming the external for being the true cause. Otherwise, smoking would be shown to be the true cause in all cases.

Another example is someone in the household acquires mononucleosis. All the family members continued to drink out of the same cups, yet only one of the family member's got sick. Why not all?

As another example, consider five children who were playing in a field of poison ivy. Three acquired it, but two did not. In fact, the one of who was most highly susceptible to this element was one of the two unaffected children. Why then would this element affect some and not others if it were the true cause? Why such inconsistency?

These inconsistencies indicate that the true cause is not the external; rather the external is the trigger that activates the internal cause. We will always be able to point fingers at external manifested things as the cause for dis-ease, because there will always be an external trigger that will provoke an internal reaction.

Dis-ease is an internal process that is triggered by external means. The external process is recognized because it is easily seen or identified, but the internal process is not so easily recognizable or understood, and that is the reason for the mistake of identifying the external as the true *cause* for dis-ease.

Dis-ease follows a process of steps and stages before it becomes evident at the biological body. Thus, dis-ease does not come out of nowhere; it has been there a long time in the making. Often we are just unaware of its presence until it reaches the physical body. Until then most are clueless to the dis-ease felt within. In fact, if it were not for dis-ease reaching the biological body and causing pain, discomfort, hindrance, etc. , we would never pay attention to the dis-ease felt within our body. Pain is the soul's message to heal. Pain is the way that the dis-ease can express its discomfort so that the soul learning can finally be heard and learned.

Once the dis-ease reaches the biological body, we need to become aware of its nature and try to understand it. We need to learn that our body is the indicator of dis-ease within. We must find the avenue the dis-ease has taken, whether it be present or long-term circumstances, feelings, thoughts and/or various states of well-being. Eventually we will be able to see the pattern that is present in our life when a certain dis-ease keeps reoccurring. Over time, we will come to understand the pattern and relationship which will allow us to see why and how it develops. And so, when we see the pattern present, we can learn to catch the dis-ease ahead of time.

Potentially catching the dis-ease at the emotional and mental stages, gives us the opportunity to find balance. The more we become aware of ourselves and our soul learnings, the better we will be able to catch dis-ease at these early stages, thus *preventing dis-ease at the biological level*. This awareness includes catching the messages from our soul through the experiences presented to us in our life for learning.

Once dis-ease reaches the biological level, a key sign to look at is the nature of the body part or organ that is faced with dis-ease. For example, consider stomach problems. We know that the stomach biologically is the digestive process. Metaphorically, stomach ailments tell us that we are having trouble digesting and accepting something in our life right now. It is not just something we ate. Remember, the stomach is the last stage to see this difficulty one is having with digesting something in their life. Having trouble digesting does not just exist at the biological body. The emotional, mental and spiritual levels are first having trouble digesting long before difficulty is ever felt at the biological level, such as in this case the stomach. Therefore by one accepting what it is in their life that they are having a hard time with, knowing that all things are divine and meant to be for a reason, the sooner the dis-ease can exist the body.

For another example, consider foot problems. Our feet allow us to take our steps to walk through life. Metaphorically, if we are having trouble with our feet, either we are having trouble taking a step long overdue or we have been taking too many steps in one direction somewhere in our life.

If we are able to identify the nature of the dis-ease by looking at the biological function and understanding it, then we can metaphorically relate it to better understand its nature. Just as when it arises at the physical body, we can pay attention to the previous circumstances, situations, thoughts, and feelings that were occurring right before the onset of the dis-ease at the biological level. These are ways to learn to identify the soul learning related to the dis-ease.

The dis-ease is present as a clear message to teach us something. We need to come to terms with the learning for the dis-ease to exit the body. Avoidance doesn't work. Truly we can't get rid of it until we acquire the soul learning. It will return to show itself time and time again. Until its purpose has been obtained, the dis-ease will continue to exist. We need to accept its presence and discover its message – soul learning.

Once we are at the point where we are learning, we will then begin to become more adaptable to the pain. The pain will not seem to bother us as much, or the symptoms may even seem to go away. This change happens because we are learning bits and pieces of our soul learning.

Later the pain or symptoms may come back to get our attention again. This reappearance means the learning is presenting itself again for further learning. We will continue to learn and strengthen our learning until we come to complete understanding. We don't need to become discouraged if the dis-ease begins to relieve or go into remission and then later returns. This is part of the healing process, just don't give up!

When the pain and symptoms re-present themselves, re-surface, it is not necessarily because we have not done any learning; we have learned in part, and now it is time to further gain the understanding needed for more learning. The dis-ease, the pain and symptoms, keep resurfacing because if the pain, *the message to heal*, did not keep coming back to remind us, we would just stop working on our soul learning.

Dis-ease cannot be avoided or dodged. It will find an avenue for expression. Our soul will magnetically align itself with the opportunity to experience the necessary learning intended for our soul. If we continue to avoid these messages we only bring ourselves more grief and pain. We must come to understand the true cause, which is the soul learning for our dis-ease. We need to face it, accept it and put this learning into application in our lives. Then, and only then will we be able to overcome the dis-ease. Whether the dis-ease is at the subtle levels, mental and emotional or at the physical body itself, when we address the cause, soul learning, we are then able to truly overcome the dis-ease.

6

POTENTIALITY vs. LIMITATIONS
POSSIBILITIES vs. IMPOSSIBILITIES

WHEN WE acquire our soul learnings they turn into our strengths, which is how we strengthen our immune system and how we advance our consciousness. We are only beginning to realize the infinite possibilities that are available to us through the advancement of our consciousness. This advancement allows us to open up and explore the infinite possibilities available to us in life. We have barely begun to tap into our potentiality as spiritual beings.

We have no idea how bound we are by our own conscious limitations. These limitations are limits we see on something as being impossible. Whatever our consciousness perceives as a limitation automatically becomes a limitation or impossibility for our entire being. We are bound by that belief, and thus we will indeed see it play as a reality in our life, because that is what we have committed to. So many of us commit to these limitations with too many things in life, thus automatically limiting them from manifesting in our lives. We no longer have to remain restricted by old mindsets, by what is known, but rather we need to jump into the unknown to prove the impossible. Anything that appears impossible seems so only because we have not yet made it possible.

Limitations surround us and constrict us to conform, often even without our conscious realization. We have no idea how held back we are, not just by our own conscious limitations, but also by the limitations of the collective consciousness, society as a whole. These conscious limitations, both by our own self-influence and by the influence of others, become limitations in our lives to us.

If our belief is not to be open to everything, than it is guaranteed that our belief will hold us back from something. If we do not see everything as possible, then the perceived impossibilities become our limitations. Thus it is important that we learn to be as open-minded as we can.

After we have learned to overcome some of our personal limitations, the conditioning from the social consciousness is the next limitation to overcome. The social consciousness is the collective norms view. The way the majority sees it becomes the standard and mindset of what is.

We are afflicted by social conscious limitations both consciously and subconsciously. Consciously, we can be aware of these limitations put on us and then either try to conform to them or struggle to overcome them. Subconsciously, we may not be aware of the limitations put on us; thus we automatically conform to what is, without really being aware of it. Therefore, we conform to what is known, without having discovered reality on our own, as our own truth.

Dis-ease is a prime example of how we are bound by limitations, whether they be personal beliefs (limitations) or society's beliefs (limitations). An example that involves society's limitations is cancer. If the world view is that when we acquire cancer, we will experience such and such, and then we die, then that is automatically what most will expect to do, and thus ultimately do. Most individuals automatically commit to that conscious limitation as their reality, not realizing that it does not have to be that way. Something is only impossible if we commit to it believing so. WE DO NOT have to die from cancer; rather we can learn from it and overcome it.

Because our mind programs our body, every thought or feeling we have goes to every cell in our body. So every time we believe something to be so, the body complies. Once we have a conscious commitment that something is impossible, for the most part it is impossible for us, until we can come to prove it different, if we are willing to try.

Individuals that have proved the impossible and overcame such dis-eases as cancer or paralysis succeeded because they did not buy into the downward spiral of limitations and impossibility. They believed it possible and indeed it was. The people who have overcome such dis-eases succeeded because they did not commit to dying, to letting the dis-ease take them over; instead they learned their soul learning and overcame the dis-ease.

If we want to change something in our reality, we must change our conscious perception of it, the way we look at it. Becoming more open to possibilities is the only way we can change the course of any action. The only way we are able to change our perception is through our experiences that prove new possibilities. *Learning to be more open-minded is one of the biggest keys to preventing and overcoming any dis-ease.* We must be willing to be open-minded to look at things other than just the way we have always seen them.

Having a mindset that is willing to begin to explore more than what is possible: The only way that we can truly advance our current state of consciousness. We must extend our current conscious view, or perspectives, and explore what is possible, opening up to new ideas. If we continue to look at what is through the same old perspective, then that is all that we will ever see.

Those who have the greatest of minds are those who look beyond what is known and search for what is possible, offering us our next breakthroughs in science, religion, medicine and life for our future generations.

7

SOUL'S ENCYCLOPEDIA OF DIS-EASESE FROM A – Z

A

ABDOMINAL CRAMPING

Cramping of any sort is a result of someone restricting and constricting energy: holding on and letting go, back and forth, with great inner conflict. They are willing, then hesitant. This puts the body in a spasmodic mode. In particular, cramping in the abdominal area relates to one who is having a hard time accepting what they are going through in their life right now. What is coming at them in life right now is more than they are quite willing or able to accept, so they question, "Can I go on?" They are having a hard time dealing with the circumstances at hand. They are having trouble with what life is dealing out to them. Although they are doing their best at trying to keep up, they are questioning whether they can.

Their soul learning is that they need to *accept* where they are at in life right now, knowing that their soul has put them right where they need to be. Instead of thinking that they can't handle what is going on and thus questioning whether they can go on, rather they need to learn to accept where they are at and what is gong on. They must remember that God does not give us more than we can handle, even though it seems like it many times.

To understand what they are having a hard time accepting, they need to trace back to what they were thinking, feeling or doing prior the onset of their abdominal cramping. They need to look at what was going on around them. Keep in mind that the longer it has been since the dis-ease appeared, the harder it will be to think back to the origin that sparked this soul learning. In other words, something they saw, heard or did or some person, place or thing triggered the soul learning of this dis-ease. Dis-ease occurs as a last attempt to get our attention, often involving pain, suffering and struggle. If we didn't get sick or have pain we would never pay attention to our bodies, ultimately denying our soul learnings.

ABSCESSES

Individuals that acquire an abscess don't feel safe expressing their own feelings within a particular situation or circumstance or to another individual. They have been carrying a specific hidden emotion that they have been harboring and concealing. This emotion has been eating away at them for some time. They have not been able to come to terms with it. Rather, it has been avoided because the individual doesn't know how to deal with it. Now it has been triggered through a particular life experience, because now is the time for it to be faced and dealt with.

The reason this emotion has not been dealt with is that the individual does not feel *safe* to express it. They don't feel safe to express and stand up for their feelings, thoughts and beliefs. These individuals lack security. This individual's soul learning is that they need to learn to feel safe to express what they truly feel.

The problem is that they don't see the purpose in expressing what they feel. They don't see how important it is for them to express their feelings. They don't see the point. Therefore, they close themselves off from dealing with these feelings. Yet, the abscess itself is stating that they can no longer continue to close themselves off from this particular emotion. They need to learn to open up their mouth and express their feelings on the particular subject, situation or person. Not only will it help them (and their abscess), it will also help the situation, person, etc. around them. Remember that each person is in the exact experience they need, so the situation or person that is present is there for a reason and needs to hear what you have to say to help them on the situation, as well as you.

If one is unable to identify the hidden emotion, then to pinpoint they will need to look at what occurred in their life just prior to the onset of this abscess to the best of their abilities. They need to trace back and look at the situations and circumstances that they were involved in prior to this onset. Then they must look at the particular feelings that arose and surfaced before and/or during these experiences. This reflection will help them to identify the particular emotion involved in the onset of the abscess. Therefore he or she is able to freely express their feelings, allowing them to overcome their abscess – soul learning.

ACIDIC STOMACH

Acidic stomach occurs when the hydrochloric acid in the stomach increases to above-normal levels. Hydrochloric acid is always present in the stomach; it is a necessary element for the metabolic breakdown during digestion. Without this acid we would not be able to digest food. We need to have a pH balance of acid and alkaline to keep our digestive system up and running, as well as indirectly helping our whole being. Problems arise when there is a sudden increase in this acid. This increase throws off the pH balance that affects all states of our being.

This increase in acid arises because the body has been informed that it needs to provide extra digestion power, so to speak. This message is sent because someone is trying too hard to digest what life has handed to them. They can't seem to quite chew this up, *accept* this, and so they try too hard. These messages sent to the brain in turn produce's more hydrochloric acid, therefore creating an acidic stomach.

The acid level in the stomach increases because the individual is taking in too much stimuli - things, thoughts, feelings, etc. - at a faster rate then they are used to handling. This overload is due to the fact that they are having trouble accepting what their soul has brought to them for learning and so they are trying too hard to accept this. This happens because they are trying to be who and where they are not.

Their soul learning is that they need to *accept who they are and where they are at in life*. They are going in vicious circles because they are having trouble accepting what has been dealt to them in life. First, they need to accept that they are having trouble and that it is OK, everyone has trouble when it comes to their learnings. From there they need to take a look at why their soul is bringing this to their attention. They need to take a look at the soul learning that is being expressed; accept it, knowing it's necessary for their souls learning; and then slowly start to adapt this learning into their character/being.

ACNE

Having acne signifies that one is having a hard time with one's self-identity. These people are bothered about their external appearance. What these individuals need to realize is that we are all unique individuals, so when we express our true self, we are not always going to be accepted by others with a positive response. Not being accepted is what is bothering these individuals. Therefore, they close off parts of themselves in their life, not letting their true self out. By keeping themselves concealed, they cause a backup of energy (clogged pores) that erupt into acne. The severity of the acne reflects how much they are not being who they truly are.

These individuals are too worried about how they look on the outside. They need to look more at what's on the inside – Who they really are. They need to focus on the principles that count in life, rather than the superficial. They are locked into rigid ways of how they should be, look and appear. It would be helpful to them to be open to some new possibilities for how to express their uniqueness. We are all divine and unique. That is what makes us so dynamic. These individuals need to let that uniqueness shine – don't smother it!

They are closing themselves off from being who they are because of some negative responses that they experienced in the past that has now created them to not be OK with their self. Their soul learning is they need to learn to continue to put themselves back out there in life being all of who they are, regardless of negative responses. They need to focus on the positive responses that they receive from being who they truly are. Over time, they will come to see that the positives outweigh the negatives. When they no longer focus on the fear of the negative response, they will come to freely express who they are, and this is how the acne will be eliminated.

ATTENTION DEFICIT DISORDER

Children who face Attention Deficit Disorder (ADD) are in great inner turmoil about themselves and where they can fit into this picture of life. They are in conflict over their inner urges about themselves in relation to life. In the external world, they see limitations and standards that they do not fit into. Therefore, they often feel lost.

Although they have eager urges, they feel they cannot express themselves, so they end up with a lot of built-up energy within and no *proper* external outlet for it. Eventually, this energy does find a way out through other outlets such as fidgeting, rebelliousness, lack of attention and misbehavior. This energy that seems misplaced is indeed misplaced, because they need to learn how to create a positive avenue for this energy through their own unique self-expression. The problem is that they don't know how to fully express and share their individual uniqueness.

The majority of people in the world are still conditioned with old ways of looking at things, often being very closed minded about new ways. They are comfortable, safe and secure with the way things are. They apply this mindset to their children, thinking that their children should follow the same path that they did, after all, it worked for them. This is not to say that the conditioned old mindset is right or wrong; rather, it has helped us to become who we are today. The point is to not let this old way of thinking hold us back from a new and different way of looking at or doing things. We don't need to let the new truths that are forming today be held back because we are stuck viewing life only through the old standards and truths.

Many children, particularly those with ADD, are more open-minded and ready for the new. Their mindsets have broken free from the old conditioned ways of thinking, and they are now having a hard time trying to find a new avenue of expression for the unique individuals that they are.

They are unable to understand how they can make a place for themselves in this world. They daydream because in their mind they can *be* themselves. This is their escape. Yet, they must realize that they need to learn how to compromise in life, to learn that things might not always be as they desire. Just because they can't exist exactly as they see fit, they are not exempted from participating in this world. They must still take advantage of what life has to offer them and be as true to themselves as they can, in as many ways as they can.

These individuals need to realize that we are all authentic, and we need to do something with our uniqueness. They need to take what they have dreamt and imagined and create it into reality. Their soul learning is that they need to bring their dreams into reality, to put them into application to the best of their ability. *Life is God's gift to us, and what we do with our life is our gift back to God.*

Since the children of today are growing in a new time and age their goals are likely to be different from those of their parents. This change is hard for many parents to understand. If the children are rebelling against the current system, it is because they are trying to break free from the old mindset to reach a new mindset, a new way of thinking and doing things. This is why many teachers have trouble working with ADD children. These teachers need new approaches to the old rhetoric. They need to put more imagination into their way of teaching. Trying to force these children to conform to the old way of thinking is unlikely to work or be of any benefit to the child or the teacher. Truly the best thing parents or teachers can do to help these children is to be more open-minded and encourage them to be *anything* they want to be, and help them figure out how they can achieve it, instead of forcing them to be something they are not.

ACQUIRED IMMUNODEFICIENCY SYNDROME

People born with immune problems have been preset right from the start with this particular soul learning, which is to *rise and take a stand* for who they are. This soul learning is passed down from generation to generation until it is acquired. This is true with all dis-eases. All those who acquire AIDS have a similar problem, yet the way in which they acquire AIDS makes a difference. Although slight, the difference still counts.

Homosexual/Bisexual: These people have come into life with a certain sexual preference that leads them to *be different* from the majority. Although it is hard being different from the majority, this gives them the opportunity that challenges them to stand up for who they truly are. This is the last attempt, a learning experience for souls who need to learn to *stand up* for themselves no matter how different they may be.

Those who *hide* and don't stand up for themselves can end up with AIDS if they don't acquire the learning. Standing for who they are and not hiding it is more of an inner battle than anything else. Not only do they not *stand* up for themselves, they *hide* their true selves from others. What they don't realize is that they only person they are truly hiding from is themselves; nothing else counts.

People that have Aids, all do this same thing, one does not have to be homosexual/bisexual, thus hiding from their sexual energy, rather one could be hiding from another part of their true self in other ways. This is why there is more than just homosexual/bisexual people that acquire this dis-ease.

Individuals who acquire AIDS from needles – drug use. First one must understand drug users (look to Drug addiction) and why they use drugs, then we can more fully understand why and how they would acquire this dis-ease through drugs. In short, people who use drugs are using them to run away from the present conditions of life instead of trying to cope. Drugs offer a newperspective on life, it makes life appear *better* than it is. Truly it is a way to run within themselves and hide, to then create their own world within themselves. In their world within they can create their own standards for living. These individuals acquire AIDS because they hide their true self as well. They deny themselves to BE in life. They desperately need to step into life – to take a stand stating I am alive, I am me, instead of trying to create an illusion that is not who they really are. This resorts back to the issue of them not feeling good enough about themselves. Many times they are homeless, where they are not seen – here again we can see how they are able to hide. As well, even with famous people; they can hide behind the performing person they are.

All others who acquire AIDS such as through a blood transfusion, etc, did not acquire this dis-ease by accident. They too are suffering from a *hidden self*.

They are not standing for themselves. To be particular would take too long to explain, yet in some regard they cannot stand up for who they really are and what they really want out of life overall, no matter what it is.

To acquire a dis-ease such as AIDS, one would have to have done a lot of hiding of who they are, to the point where the individual has stopped fighting to make a stand that they even exist in life. As a result the body does the same; every cell begins to show the same pattern. When one gives up the fight for who they truly are, trouble is sure to arise. The hope at this point is that in this desperate attempt for their life, they will learn *how to fight* for themselves and their life, how to stand up for who they truly are and how to let themselves speak in new ways – to let their unique soul be heard.

ALCOHOLISM

These individuals have an inner conflict about what reality actually is vs. what reality is to them. This conflict is both within themselves and about themselves in relation to life. Their focus is on a reality that is not as it currently is. They are caught up in their world, seeing things as *they see them.*

They spend a lot of time thinking about another reality to avoid this one. In their reality, the way they see themselves and life is acceptable. The altered state provided by alcohol allows them to exist in their reality. In this slightly altered state the world seems safe to them, and often this is the only way that many can tolerate functioning in daily life routines. This altered state allows them to look at and face life more easily, because stone cold reality is too hard for them to deal with.

Their soul learning is that they need to realize that they cannot escape what is, even if it is not to their liking. Running, which is what they are doing by trying to escape this reality, or it will be passed on to their children; future generations to learn the consequences of this lack of discipline. Acquiring this learning in this generation is the way to help our future generations. This is true will all dis-eases. It is better to face what is and accept it, instead of disregarding it or avoiding it, because ultimately we can't avoid what is meant to be. Doing this will save us a lot of grief.

These individuals must learn to ask themselves, "Do I have self- discipline?" This requires them to take a good look at all areas in their life where there may be a lack of self-discipline, and then learn to discipline themselves in those areas. They must learn to discipline themselves to refrain from escaping, by learning different ways to cope with this reality and rather be responsible by facing this reality. They must accept that there are rules and regulations that they will indeed have to follow, some harder than others. They need to spend more time looking back and remembering the blessings they do have in their life, whether few or many. It's also important for them to realize that life has balances: with any up, there is always a down etc.

For these individuals, a good statement for them to say to themselves while they continue to work on their soul learning would be:

God grant me the strength to accept my path in life, through the bad and good. God grant me the courage not only to help myself, but also to help others. God grant me the wisdom to know how to apply myself appropriately in all situations in my life:when to honor myself for who I am and when it's time to make changes within myself.

ALLERGIES

An allergy is a response by the body's immune system to a substance, situation, circumstance or person that the individual is currently having trouble adapting to within their environment. Understand that not only do we have allergic reactions to substances; we also have allergic reactions to situations, circumstances and people.

Let's take a brief minute to talk about how our immune system works. Although it is called the fighting system, it is really our adaptation system. We are not trying to fight off anything; rather, we are trying to adapt our bodies to something new and unfamiliar. Therefore, we need to learn how to adapt to it, by slowly coping through it. This indeed is how we acquire our immunities.

The body must acquire immunity to allergens, and the only way this is happen's is by coping through it and learning how to adapt to it. This is why it is important for us to not avoid the particular substance, circumstances, situations and people that we have allergic reactions to. Rather, we must learn slowly to adapt to them. From a physical point of view, the theory behind allergy shots is the same. Deeper yet, we need to slowly re-expose ourselves to these substances, circumstances, situations and people that triggered this allergic reaction in order to learn how to cope through it by coming to terms with it. By avoiding the things that we are allergic to, we will never get the opportunity to acquire the immunity for them.

These individuals like to avoid things. They run from their soul learning. Ultimately, they fear having to be reminded of the learning that is present in the particular substance, circumstances, situations or person that they have an allergic reactions to, because then they have to face what they are trying to avoid.

The reason they avoided the learning in the first place is because they are having a hard time seeing a fix for the situation, person, circumstance, etc. The deeper problem is that they don't know how to deal with it, so they try to avoid it. Even though they don't know how to deal with it, this is exactly what the individual must learn to do in order to adapt to these certain substances, situations, circumstances or people. This is their soul learning. They must face it and deal with it by learning to cope through it one step at a time.

ALZHEIMER'S DIS-EASE

Alzheimer's dis-ease arises after years of overuse of the function of recalling information from the memory bank, thereby causing a disconnection to the hippocampus (memory bank). When this happens, one is unable to retrieve the memory stored there. It's not that the memory is gone; the person just cannot get to it. Over time, this leads to one not being able to retrieve other basic skills, such as concentration; communication; awareness of time, space, personality; and proper muscle function. All of this leads to the idea that one has worn out their primitive cognitive system due to an overload.

Individuals that face this dis-ease are individuals who have spent too much time in the past concentrating on keeping themselves in check with everything. Their mind never quits it is always has to assure itself about its actions and reactions. Such individuals never feel completely sure or safe, even in the safest of places. They carry a constant unprotected feeling within them. They don't like feeling exposed, so they are constantly on guard, constantly seeking concealment. They are very uptight and tense people. This mode of being has led them to burn out their ability to recall memories. Now, at this stage of the process of this dis-ease they can no longer worry and go over and over everything to make sure there is safety; they are now exposed.

Although they don't look very consciously alert in the severer stages, they are still alert and alive inside, experiencing this abundant exposure that they can no longer conceal. Every time a new experience comes up that they can't remember, they feel the exposure within – at that moment. So they experience constant new shockers, being caught off guard every time they are unable to remember something.

It is best to catch this learning in the early stages by becoming OK with exposing, one self, instead of being on guard all the time. Their soul learning is to quit worrying about having to be on top of things, (or look as if they are). They need to realize that nothing in life is going to be completely and permanently safe – in fact it is only by going through *unsafe* circumstances in our life that we can learn how to feel safe.

The more one learns to become OK with exposing themselves, with revealing their faults and weaknesses, the less the symptoms of the dis-ease will persist. If we get more worried, like when were losing our memory, we shouldn't become fixated on it, but rather be OK that we forgot it. The harder we try for it to not happen, the more it will. Rather, understand it's happening to expose us – to catch us off guard - so that we can learn to be OK, coping with not only our strengths but also our weaknesses and faults being exposed. This soul learning teaches us that it's OK to be exposed and safe at the same time. Thus, the more we become comfortable with this idea, the less this dis-ease will proceed in a worse direction.

ANEMIA

Individuals with anemia suffer from such symptoms as feeling weak and becoming easily fatigued and run down. These individuals have a weak inner self. Not much is expressed, and what little that is expressed, is often not the whole truth. They don't express all of who they are. They keep that hidden deep within. What we see on the outside is not all of who they really are on the inside. They even try to fool themselves.

Their soul learning is that they need to learn to let themselves come out like a tiger with all of who they are, fully expressing their truths, feelings, thoughts and beliefs about life. This will in turn help them to become stronger with who they are, instead of keeping their self-hidden within. By not letting themselves out, they are denying themselves the chance to get what they need out of life. In essence, as they deny who they are, their blood, their life force, suffers until they again learn to honor that hidden self, letting it be heard.

ANOREXIA

Anorexic people are perfectionists. This dis-ease is seen predominately in women who are always striving for the best in everything. When they cannot live up to the standards that they themselves have created, then there is a problem. Understand that the expectations that they create for themselves are far greater than any expectations that society or anybody else could possibly have for them.

They think that the only way to prove their worth is to meet these high expectations. How they measure their self-worth is by their accomplishments. When they feel that they have failed in any sense, they take it very deep and hard. They start to punish themselves, which turns into self-destruction. Denying themselves food is commonly an internal punishment for them not being worthy, in their own eyes. The focus for helping these individuals should not be on food itself; rather, their focus should be on building their self-esteem, and then they will accept food. It will not work the other way around. They need to work on the true problem, which is in this case is *lack of self-worth.*

In the case of anorexia, it is not just that they don't feel that they do good enough; rather, the deeper issue is that they feel they are not good enough. Their self-worth needs to be built up. Unfortunately, it's not enough just to tell them that they are worthy and then they will be; rather, they must experiences it and believe it themselves.

The soul learning for these individuals is to move away from focusing so much on what they didn't accomplish or how what they did accomplish wasn't as perfect as they thought it should be and to move toward seeing the worth in what they did indeed accomplish. They need to spend less time judging their outer self and take more time looking at the good within their self.

ANXIETY

Anxiety is a state in which someone feels very edgy, uncomfortable, unsettled and uncertain. They can never feel quite satisfied. People who suffer from anxiety are people who have an *on-the-go* lifestyle. Their inner feeling of uncertainty towards life is motivated by their lifestyle. This uncertainty exists because they are lacking the knowledge to approach certain situations or circumstances in their life. This lack causes them to feel very uncomfortable and edgy in life, a state that can overtime lead to anxiety.

Often these individuals do a lot of responding. It makes them feel better if they respond. They are always going, going and going, like nervous energy just scattering all about. This behavior happens because they lack the understanding in their mind about certain circumstances or situations in their life, so their minds continue to go on and on looking for this understanding that they do not have. This often leads to one not being able to go to sleep or stay asleep at night (See Insomnia).

These individuals need to learn to *let go and let God!* They need to realize that there are certain things in their life that they have control of and they can do something about, while there are other things in their life that they do not have control of and they must learn to let these things go. They need to stop wasting energy by worrying about things they don't have control over. There is no more that they can do, because there is no more that they are supposed to do: it's out of their hands and in God's. God has a divine plan for all things.

The soul learning for these individuals is to learn to RELAX and let go of the things that they have no control of. They need to try to force themselves to NOT go and do – even if it requires taking some type of sedative or using an alternative means to relax, such as meditation. This will help them to be able to take time and evaluate things in order to gain the knowledge they need before they can properly respond in life. Having this knowledge will eliminate the anxiety for them because then they will have an underlying sense of security.

ARTERIOSCLEROSIS

Individual who blocks energy from freely flowing in their life can create this blockage in the arteries. This arises because they have avoided dealing with too many situations in their life. They have spent too much time trying to figure things out in life, predominately from a mental perspective, with little to no emotional involvement. They don't allow emotions to come in, let alone be felt.

They often pretend that emotions don't even exist.

Their soul learning is that they need to learn to deal with the feelings that they are trying to avoid. They need to confront the situations in their life that they are ignoring, by expressing their feelings about it. By blocking themselves off from feeling in life, they are stopping emotions, which stops energy (blood) from freely flowing.

They need to stop closing off their heart, which is an emotional center in the brain, from coming in as well as going out. They must open their heart and wake up to their feelings, even to other's feelings. *It's OK – safe to express who you are.* We are all unique individuals here to share with each other our own individual uniqueness.

ARTHRITIS – OSTEOARTHRITIS

This dis-ease most often starts when one gets older, although this condition is not limited to older people. This dis-ease develops when an individual stops giving them self what they need to keep their body going – his/her purpose!Because they are getting older he/she no longer thinks that they have a purpose. They think that they don't count in life, thus they can no longer be productive.

Arthritis commonly affects us so that we cannot move easily for ourselves to *do* – to produce. This impairment develops out of the individuals fear about whether or not they can live up to the standards of life. Thus they inhibit their own selves from *doing* in order to avoid directly facing the fact that they truly may not be able to do what they used to do.

This perspective is why this dis-ease most commonly affects us as we get older. Those who have acquired this dis-ease, both the elderly and others that are not older, tend to start giving up in life. They begin to let life take them over, and they no longer fight for their place in life. They sit back and lose touch, because they think that they no longer *fit* in life. They question their abilities to perform.

People in this situation need to realize that they can always still live up to life. They must realize that they only need to adapt to a new way of doing things. Yes, what they do may change. What they need to realize is that life is about change, about going through the cycles presented to them. They don't need to stop going through the cycles of life just because they do not fill the positions that they used to or want to. There are many new positions still out there for them. There is always a place for them to fit.

The body's joints allow for flexibility, so stiff joints reflect one's inflexibility to bend and adapt to new situations that life brings. Someone with arthritis gets stuck in the mindset that they can't *do*. But the fact is that they can do – and they need to do. The more they avoid participating, the worse the arthritis will get. They need to find new ways to still do things and activities, and to learn to stop limiting themselves. Limiting themselves is the last they need to be doing.

The soul learning is they need to realize that they do count, no matter what they do or do not do. Life does indeed have a place for them, as long as they continue to participate in life. By not giving up on them self, there will always be a place for them in life. Someone who never gives up on them self will always find a place in life.

ASTHMA

An individual who acquires asthma is emotionally sensitive. When emotional upsets arise, an asthma attack can easily be triggered. They begin to gasp for air, trying to catch another breath. They question if they will be able to handle it, make it through. They don't know if they are going to be able to confront or deal the situation at hand. The outcome depends on how emotionally overwhelming the experience was for them.

Asthmatics have a hard time dealing with uncomfortable situations. They don't like to confront problems or stir up any emotions. They would rather say nothing than create waves. They prefer to keep their feelings hidden deep within about many matters. They literally try to avoid the feelings that arise when they are faced with an uncomfortable situation, because they think that they aren't capable of dealing with the situation. What they don't realize is that by not confronting and dealing with the situations that life presents to them, they are actually denying themselves their very essence - who they truly are: body, mind, spirit and heart! They need to learn that we are *all* unique individuals, with different perspectives that we all must learn to offer to life by confronting and dealing with life situations. They need to remember that God doesn't give us more than we can handle.

Their soul learning is that they need to learn to express their feelings in life regardless of how uncomfortable it is, or whose feelings may be disturbed. This is essential; otherwise they will continue to deny themselves the breath of life. They must learn not to avoid their feelings. They need to remember that these feelings exist for a reason, and they need to take a look at that reason. Avoiding situations, circumstances and people that are too emotionally overwhelming will only create more and different experiences for them to face. They will continue to have experiences that provoke their feelings, until they learn to express their true feelings. After they realize that they need to act upon their feelings, eventually they will express their feelings appropriately when all situations arise in their life. Expressing one's true feelings is the key to releasing and preventing the onset of asthma attacks.

ATHEROSCLEROSIS

These individuals tend to be very tense people. They have a hard time accepting change easily. Typically, a person who develops atheroscherosis doesn't allow things to happen freely in life, just taking or accepting things as they are. If things are not as they desire they can become very resentful and closed-minded, thus blocking energy from freely flowing in their life. However, they don't see themselves as close-minded; they see it as staying on track. They look at things only from their perspective, instead of being open-minded and seeing others' perspectives, therefore opening up to new ideas.

Such an individual is unhappy deep within about some situation or person. They have a backup of old, stored emotions and hurts having to do with this area of their life. They have not yet been able to let go of these now *resentful* emotions, and so these feelings have stayed stuck. The result is a back up of energy leading to atherosclerosis.

Their soul learning is that they need to learn to release things by forgiving within their hearts. They can do this by understanding that we all do the best we can at the time. They will be able to release their hurts through understanding the cause that has been keeping them so stuck in this state of resentment. As we forgive, we release the burden of resentment, through the understanding of it we come to be more open-minded to others' perspectives to help us see and learn many new things in life.

ATHLETES FEET

Athletes are prone to acquire this dis-ease, but unathletic types often get it too. In either case, these individuals are *questioning themselves and their ability to perform.* They question whether or not they count as a person or even to the team, in the case of athletes. Individuals that acquire this dis-ease are feeling that their time has passed with the position or sport that they are in. They are now letting themselves fade away. Individuals that acquire athlete's foot are or have been taken over by the game of life. They are falling between the cracks of life, and are now dealing with a sense of a *lost identity.*

These people aren't getting out of the *game of life* what they used to get. They have lost power in their position within life and are now just going through the motions. Their soul learning is that they need to either regain their position, coming back into the game of life even stronger, or find a new place or position for themselves that will again inspire them to participate in the game of life.

B

BACK PROBLEMS
(LOWER. MIDDLE AND UPPER BACK)

The spine indicates the backbone or structure of the person, which is related to their composure. Back problems occur because an individual is placing an enormous amount of pressure on their self to perform. These expectations *to do* enables them to feel good in their mind. Having this state of mind - of taking on so much, and thus over exerting the body - enables them to live up to their expectations of themselves. This attitude induces a lot of worry and pressure. The pressure and worrying are constantly present because they are always questioning if they can now perform what they have put themselves up to doing. When they don't measure up to these expectations, then they feel that they have failed in some sense and so their composure goes out of alignment, thus literally their structure, their back, goes out of place.

Because there are so many different soul learning's for every individual, the back can become out of alignment, from mildly to severely, by many different means, depending on the individual's unique soul learnings.

LOWER BACK

People who have lower back problems are into *perfection* as a source or evaluation of their structure and composure in life. These people are not just into pressure to perform; the performance must be perfect – the highest level of expectations. They cannot stand imperfection in themselves and do their very best to conceal it. Imperfection makes them feel less about themselves, as if they are not good enough. Because they expect so much of themselves, they don't realize just how excessive these expectations are, thus they expect too much of their bodies, trying so hard to reach this level of perfection. When they are not able to live up to this level of perfection in their minds, then they think and feel that they have failed. *They are not happy with themselves.* Therefore their structure and composure have been shaken, causing the back to become out of alignment.

The soul learning for these people is that they need to realize that everything is perfect as it is. It is not about us looking perfect, but rather that we're already perfect exactly the way we are. We are all very unique individuals, each perfect as we are.

MIDDLE BACK

People who have middle back problems are into *capacity*. These people *over invest* themselves into too many things. They are not hesitant enough. They need to think before responding in specific areas of life. Because they feel that they get no support, they often "take on the world" themselves out of spite, trying to make up for the perceived lack. They are very critical of themselves. They fear a letdown in their structure, discovering something that they can't do. To them, this means failure, and failure brings fear of rejection. They fear rejection because they think they are not good enough. If they are not able, then they are not good enough. This is how such individuals measure things in their life.

The soul learning for these individuals is to learn to not over invest oneself: beginning by learning to say *no*. What we can and cannot do is not a measure of our worth. As long as one is doing what they are truly capable of, that is all that counts.

UPPER BACK

People who have upper back problems put too much *pressure and responsibility* on themselves, believing they are capable of handling it. They take in so much energy, stressing them self out with this overload, and just let it build. When the energy builds to an excess, it eats away at them, causing pain. They handle every situation in life by taking it on – and in. By storing all of these problems, the energy gets stuck in the upper back. Overtime, the build- up of this energy causes the back to slip out of place.

The soul learning for these individuals is to learn to release the pressure by accepting responsibility only to the limit of what is comfortable for them. They will be less tense and more able to enjoy doing what they want, instead of feeling over pressured by an overload of responsibility.

BALDNESS

Over a period of time of living in a state of unhappiness with where one is at in life, a man or woman begins to loose their hair. They are not happy with what they have done and who they have become. They blame themselves for the unhappy picture they see them self in, and they harbor guilt over what they should have done. Their sense of pride and self-worth is low. Their status is not as they want it to be. At this point they begin to feel hopeless. They give up because they feel as if the joy is gone from their life – it's too late for everything. Unfortunately, such men or woman end up wallowing in self-pity and use that as an excuse to not go forward in life. They usually just end up letting themselves go and so the hair begins or continues to go.

The soul learning for these individuals is they need to realize that, yes, they have put themselves where they are. They have put themselves not only into the unhappy and unpleasant experiences, but also into the happy and good times, and those are what they especially need to look at. They need to focus more on the good and happy moments they have had, instead of staying stuck on what they don't have. In their minds, they don't think it's possible to be happy with where they are at in life. They need to open up to new possibilities by diving back into life again and looking to see the vast possibilities available for them right now, right where they are. They need to rediscover who they are and what they want to do in life. This may be something they didn't have time to do before. Nonetheless, they need to find where they can fit in this picture of life. There is a divine place in life for everyone.

BLADDER PROBLEMS

Someone who acquires bladder problems has a weak will. The bladder becomes weak because their desire towards life is not what it used to be. They are not nearly as eager to jump into things as they once were. As their will to live continues to become weaker, the bladder becomes weakened. They have let go of their control over the natural happenings in life. "How it goes it goes", and the bladder follows the same tune – *it goes when it goes*, and not necessarily at an appropriate or planned time.

Their soul learning is to learn to let go of things that they really don't have control over and start strengthening their will about the things they can control. It's time to get back into the game of life with eagerness. Standing firm for their truths will help to lift their spirits and strengthen their will. To strengthen the bladder, one must strengthen their own will to live and to get back into life and get things in order.

BLEEDING
(IN GENERAL)

The blood in the body is a reflection of the *energy* level in the body. Someone who bleeds is having trouble allowing a proper flow of energy - blood - out of the body. This is because they cannot let things in their life - freely run their course. These individuals are the type that restrains their energy. When their surroundings are unpleasant, they often refrain from participating. They hold back. They feel very *unsafe* about participating in life. A lot of their fear is the fear of the *result*, because in life is not always a "sure thing. "Therefore, life feels unsafe. They cannot deal with that very well because overall they fear *rejection*. They hold back so they don't have to face this. The problem is that they have held themselves back too many times. The learning catches up with them. Eventually, it builds and bursts. How much one bleeds depends on how much was built up.

Bleeding means the person has been too restrictive. They need to become more free and open to the outcomes and results of things in life. Their soul learning is that they must face life regardless of the results and overcome the *rejection* they fear.

BLOOD CLOTS

The true nature of blood clots metaphorically speaking, is to form a *block*. An individual with blood clots, blocks the life force (blood) within themselves from freely flowing. They literally stop the energy, which in this case is their emotions, from freely coming and going. When the give and take are no longer equal, then the blood is unable to move freely, and it stops and clots.

There is a situation in their life that they are not confronting and dealing with, either recent, if the blood clots are recent, or a long-term situation, if the blood clots have been around for awhile. In other words, either there is a particular situation they are choosing not to emotionally deal with or confront, or in their life overall they don't emotionally deal with and confront situations.

These individuals tend to look at things from a mental perspective too much. They think they have things figured out. They are not going to face certain emotions. Their avoidance technique is to not let their emotions in to be felt. They try to pretend the emotions aren't there. Yet, they are there and ultimately can't be avoided. They do come in to be felt no matter how hard they try not to let them affect them.

The reason that these individuals with blood clots have this problem is because they don't know how to confront difficult situation(s). Ultimately, they suppress their feelings about it. Because they don't know how to deal with these feelings, they just try to avoid them. Yet these emotions still exist and they can't be ignored forever. They demand to be heard. The result is clots.

Their soul learning is to allow their feelings to freely be felt and expressed. Once they learn to more freely express their feelings by confronting situations and dealing with them, the blood will no longer clot and will begin to freely flow through the body again.

BLOOD PRESSURE
HIGH AND LOW

The flow of the blood in the body works in a harmonious way. The blood is monitored as the pressure of blood flow going in and coming out from the heart. Looking at it from another perspective, these are thoughts and feelings coming in and going out. Blood goes in and out of our heart, just as thoughts and feelings go in and out of our lives, some that we express, some that we over-express and others that we keep hidden deep within.

There is a difference in the significance of the blood coming out of the heart, compared to the blood going to the heart. The rate of blood coming out, represented by the systolic pressure, is directly related to thoughts and feelings being expressed. On the other hand, the diastolic pressure reflects to the rate of blood coming in, which is related to our thoughts and feelings coming in. This is in relation to the emotions that an individual receives and feels.

When someone's blood pressure is low, the rate of emotional energy flowing in and out is slow. This can cause one to be emotionally aloof or standoffish in receiving emotions, as well as in giving or expressing their thoughts and feelings to others. When someone's blood pressure is too high, the rate of emotional energy flowing in and out is fast, with too many thoughts and feelings (emotions) coming in at one time as well as going out. The state of the systolic and diastolic pressures tells us whether there is an overload of emotions pouring out (high systolic pressure) or an overload of emotions that we are receiving, that is coming in (high diastolic pressure).

In our society the most common problem is having high systolic and/or diastolic pressure rather than low, therefore we will discuss the specifics of high systolic and diastolic pressure:Individuals who have more trouble with the diastolic pressure being too high have an overload of emotions coming inthat they are avoiding because they are having trouble with the learnings. They don't even want to pay attention to them. Their motto is that if they don't feel, they don't have to deal. They need to stop trying to shut off their emotions and rather face and deal with them. The old myth that tells us "don't open up to emotions because they're signs of weakness is really telling us don't use a big part of our brain. "How ridiculous!These individuals don't realize how important it is for us to open up to our emotions. They need to appropriately express their thoughts and feelings with every situation, person, place or thing that they cross paths with in life. This is why the situation exists, for the learning. While on the other hand, when the systolic pressure that is too high these people are over responsive. They feel, therefore they respond. They need to take more time and figure things out before they confront a situation or just deal with it.

The soul learning for this dis-ease is to bring the blood pressure into balance. To do this, one must have a balance of emotional energy flowing in and out properly; not too little expression, or not too much expression one way or the other.

BREAST LUMPS

Women who have breast lumps, whether benign or malignant, are facing a problem with "lost identity". After an extended period of time of not receiving as much attention (from themselves or others) as they used to, a woman may begin to lose herself. They feel as if they could be lost in the cracks of life and nobody would notice. They begin to ask "Am I noticed?"Attention is not being focused on them causing them to question who they are as a women.

These women feel lost in the crowd. They are ones who are often willing to put others before themselves and neglect their own feelings. This makes them lose themselves after a while. When we store or stuff our own feelings for the sake of another's, we begin to store who we are as a person. In other words, we push away "who we are," as if our feelings don't even count. Since the breast is a strong representation of the female energy, this is a common place for the problem to "seed" or show, since the real problem is female identity: the lack of exposure of the feminine self.

Acquiring this dis-ease within this area of the body brings attention to a women – especially to her feminine self. It brings not only her own attention, so that she can see it, but also the attention of those around her. It makes them wake up and give her the time and space that she does need as a women. In the case of a men who have breast lumps it's the same basic learning which is the feminine aspect within themselves (as we all have both feminine and masculine sides within each of us whether we are female or male) and their feelings and needs not being met, and so they lose their identity.

The soul learning for those with breast lumps is that they need to acknowledge that their feminine self needs to be exposed, in order for their needs to be expressed and met. They need to realize that we are all here to help each other, but we must not forget about our own needs. For these individuals, it's about really learning to get in touch with that feminine aspect of their self, that missing part of the self as a whole. It's a matter of learning to become aware of these feminine needs and not forgetting to acknowledge them in the midst of acknowledging others' needs.

BROKEN BONES

When someone breaks a bone, it is related to the fact that they were overreacting to a particular situation. They were too responsive to something. Rather than just sitting back and waiting to see how things would work out, they were too quick to act without much thinking.

What their soul learning is, is they need to sit back and carefully choose their options in life. These individuals are trying to do too much, to catch everything. They tend to think that they can *handle it all*. This is their way to *prove* themselves, so as to appear on top of things. And, well they got caught in a situation that they couldn't handle, so they *got busted*. These individuals need to learn that they cannot do it all, nor do they have to do it all to prove their self worth.

BRONCHITIS

Those who acquire this chronic condition have developed it over an extended period of time, some over lifetimes. In other words, this is a long-standing issue that has built to point of bronchitis because a soul is living with certain emotions and not dealing with them.

These individuals make avoidance of disturbing or bothered feelings a way of life. They avoid confronting situations that require them to express their feelings. These individuals must learn that everybody has feelings and has a right to them. Feelings are not wrong, nor should they be ignored. Denying our feelings is denying a part of who we are. This is sure to lead to dis-ease.

It is also important for such people to not get caught up in *worrying* about the results of having to confront situations in their life, such as hurting somebody else's feelings or creating waves (at least that's the way they see the result). This is very hard for them to do. They want peace. Yet they don't realize that to have peace outside, we must first have peace within ourselves. Reaching this understanding requires them to come to terms with their feelings, recognize them and then learn how to express them.

Their soul learning is that when difficult situations arise they need to learn to confront them by expressing their feelings. If they continue to keep their feelings stuffed within, they will continue to have bronchitis.

The best thing that they can do now is to start speaking up as new situations arise that create disturbing and bothersome feelings. They need to learn to confront the situation or person here and now; it doesn't work to let it go and wait for "maybe another time. "The task only gets harder the longer it's delayed.

BRUISE

Someone who tends to bruise easily is one who is being emotionally fragile. This fragility shows through on the body. The skin is the part of our body that protects our inner organs so skin that is easily disrupted is a sign that the individual is getting disrupted within. Emotionally they are not able to protect themselves. A discoloration of the skin is a sign of a big disturbance or sensitivity within.

Frequent bruises show that the person is not being careful enough to protect their own body and being. They need to learn to get more in contact within themselves as well as what is going on around them. This obliviousness indicates that the person is not in connection with themselves, their own needs (feelings and thoughts). If they remain unaware, then they are unable to protect themselves, and therefore continue to remain emotionally fragile. The soul learning for such individuals is that they need to become more in touch with their feelings and thoughts and become more aware of themselves and their own inner needs.

BUNIONS

Our feet metaphorically represent the steps we take in life. People that have bunions on their feet are individuals that are having a problem with their walk through life. They can't see a place where they fit in this world. These individuals are having trouble seeing what they should be doing, so thus they "hold back" energy from *going forward*, in the case of this dis-ease, resulting in the energy lodging within their feet. They feel very "unsafe" to participate in life without this placement, therefore they become unwilling to participate by taking the steps they need to. This is because they don't see themselves fit. Ultimately, they hold their energy back from walking though life, thereby in this case creating bunions. This is very common among older individuals. At this time in their lives many face the dilemma where they no longer see themselves fit in life. Thus, they stop participating; ultimately *doing* in life.

What these individuals need to realize for their soul learning is that they don't have to know where they fit ahead of time, before they participate. Rather, they just need to recognize *who they are* and focus on participating just as they are. They will then find that they automatically have a fit and are safely able to participate in life.

BURSITIS

Bursitis causes congested energy within the shoulder area. An individual with bursitis is at a point where they are resistant to life. They are not willing to let things just happen. They are holding themselves back because they don't know what to expect. They feel *unsafe* because of a recent situation that they experienced, and are again experiencing, in which they had to face the fear of *rejection* again. This ruffles them up. Because of such recurring unpleasant situations they are holding back their energy for fear of getting rejected again. They are in fear of having to face this rejection all over again. Therefore, they are *holding them self back* from participating in life. They are unwilling to risk themselves, because they are unsure of the outcome. Such individuals are, as well, *resistant* to bending to the situations at hand in their life. They are being inflexible; thus their joints, which represents one's flexibilities, will be affected.

They need to look to the time when this disorder arose to determine the situation or circumstance that they were rejected and understand why this happened to them. Their soul learning is to move through their fear of rejection and take the risk. They need to take a look at the learnings to be gained in all situations in their life, becoming more open-minded and learning how to make some adjustments in their character by becoming more flexible in their lives. They need to look at the situations at hand and face them, instead of holding energy back and letting it build.

C

CANCER

Overall individuals who acquire cancer develop such a toxic dis-ease because they have been carrying toxic feelings inside over a long period of time about certain experience(s) of the past. These toxic feelings, such as guilt and anger, are harboring within them. This guilt and anger from the past just sits inside them, with no way out, or no answer in their mind to make it better. As a result they lack inner peace. Therefore, the toxic feeling just stays there and festers, eventually causing the self to attack itself, which is seen in the body as the cells beginning to attack each other.

The soul learning resides in this guilt that they have over things that they wish they could have done, or things they should not have done, in their past. What they don't realize is at the place and the time of the occurrences, *they did the best they could at that time.* We all really do our best. Yes, there are times when we could do better, but in general we all try to do the best that we can. These individuals need to forgive themselves and others over the past, realizing that they did the best they could as well as others at the time.

We don't realize how important it is that we allow our feelings to get out to really express who we are by bringing them to the surface and not letting them fester within. We need to make peace with our feelings, although sometimes it may seem like this is impossible to do. If we don't find ways to deal with these hurtful feelings by letting these past hurts go and taking what we can learn from them, then we are going to let them kill us. Whether they be hurtful feelings towards our self or others, they will eat us away, from within. Depending on the degree of toxic emotions is how quickly the cancer will progress.

The soul learning is that by having active cancer within us, we realize the preciousness of life and how important living is. *The past is the past*: let it go, so that we can go on in life, instead of staying stuck with the anger and guilt that stems from such deep hurt. We need to look to these emotional hurts, discover our learnings from them and stop this self-destructive path that we have been on. Remember, for new things to come into our lives we must let go of the old. We can start by letting go of all these emotional hurts, by learning to understand them and come to terms with them, so that they no longer hold us back. Life's too precious and short to waste our time and energy feeding these negative emotions. We need to learn to release these toxic feelings by expressing them from deep within. It's time to let go!

CANDIDASIS

Candidasis involves an upset of the normal flora of candida within the body. These individuals are facing some self-disappointment. They have just gone through a situation or circumstance in which they were disappointed within themselves. They felt like they failed in some sense, as if they were not able to keep up with the standards that they set up for themselves. All of this revolves around one's perception of oneself, the perception of not being able to do what one thought one could or should do. Such individuals perceive themselves as failures and with that comes disappointment and disgust.

These individuals' soul learning is to realize that their high standards are so unrealistic that nobody could measure up to them. Once they come to see the foolishness of the unrealistic standards that they have put on themselves, they can stop judging themselves so harshly, and they won't have to live in a state of disappointment and disgust.

CARPAL TUNNEL SYNDROME

This dis-ease is an inflammation of the nerve in the carpal tunnel (wrist), which causes nerve dysfunction, pain and weakness. Those who acquire this syndrome are individuals who have spent a lot of time trying to force things to work as they wish. These people put a lot of effort in trying to *change* things. They do this in an attempt to avoid a lot of things that they would rather not deal with, but which they indeed need to deal with. This is a defense mechanism they use to catch things ahead of time, so that they do not have to face what could be an unwanted result. This action is stimulated because the individual had a past learning, triggered by a past negative emotional experience that they do not want to have to face again. They are always going and doing so they do not have any time to deal with the past learning that they are trying so hard to avoid. To them this is a full proof method for catching anything that might be coming their way. Basically, they are living *on guard*. They do this as a safeguard (they think), so that they do not have to allow anything to trigger these emotions related to their past.

Such individuals need to change to a style of living where they live life as it comes, not trying to be one step ahead as a defense mechanism. The character of this syndrome is that it physically stops people from taking matters into their own hands, so that they will learn how to deal emotionally. This syndrome stops their ability to go and push and do things too quickly. They must learn to slow down and take or face what life has to offer them.

Hands deal with what we are currently involved in, our immediate circumstances in life. Individuals with this dis-ease over force the current circumstances in their life in attempts to avoid the past. Their soul learning is to realize that they do not have control over everything. *The only thing we really need to have control over is ourselves.* These individuals need to learn to just let things happen, because what is meant to be will be. They are going to happen anyway and we are not going to be able to stop or avoid them.

CATARACTS

Cataracts develop often later in life, when individuals first begin to lose sight of where they are going and what life has left to offer them. These individuals are dim with possibilities of what the future might hold for them, if anything. Because they are having a hard time *seeing* what will come to be, they avoid spending time looking into their future. They just exist stuck, taking things only day by day without any further goals or aspirations.

Over time, when someone looks at life this way, a cloudy film forms over the eye (retina), because that is exactly their outlook on life – cloudy. They can't see the possibilities of what can be for them, and they are beginning to lose hope for any place in life for themselves. As this condition gets worse, it can lead to full-fledged blindness. Then they can no longer see any possibilities in life.

The best suggestion is to catch this condition promptly. The soul learning is that they need to get out of the box, out of the constricting way they look at life. Instead of being the realist, they must try being the opportunist or optimist.

They need to open up to new possibilities, ideas, different ways to look at life, no longer limiting them self to viewing life in only one way.

CELLULITE

Individuals who have cellulite are not emotionally satisfied. This is not because somebody else is not fulfilling them emotionally, but rather because they themselves are not emotionally satisfied with themselves. Individuals that create cellulite are those that particularly can't accept who they are as a person, so they block off receiving emotions (love) from themselves, ultimately because they don't feel worthy.

The skin is the part of the body that *protects* the internal organs. Fat is a sign that the individual is trying to protect their sensitive parts, hiding their emotions. Fat surfacing under the skin is stating that there is a conflict going on between *trying* to protect them self and truly being *able* to protect them self, thus it is showing through. Their attempt at weight as a shield of protecting is not working.

This individual's soul learning is that they truly need to work on facing their own needs that are not being addressed. They need to learn to identify what they are not satisfied with, and realize that we all have a great uniqueness – let that shine, don't shield it!

CEREBRAL PALSY

When a child is born with such a dis-ease, the dis-ease indicates genetically that their soul in the past has been very resistant to this growth. They are born as they are because they have not chosen to learn and grow. So, they came into life with this dis-ease activated right from the start, to allow them the opportunity to acquire the skills to *want* to grow and continue forward. This is the case with many dis-eases: if the soul learning has been in process a long time – and resisted a long time through generations the individual will be born with the dis-ease.

These individuals are questioning *"who am I?"* because they have not yet found that out. They have not had the learning and growth to know and discover their identity. These children's soul learning is they need to learn to grow in life, to discover themselves. They need to jump into life, instead of letting it pass them by. Such a dis-ease makes an impact upon them, to make them want to learn. When you have this dis-ease you cannot stay stagnant. This makes you learn in order to adapt in life. This teaches the soul how to learn and the importance of learning.

CHEST COLDS
(SEE ALSO CONGESTION)

Individuals who acquire a chest cold have built up emotions over a particular situation that they are not willing to confront. Something has come about that has disturbed them and they have been trying to avoid their feelings about it. Sure, they have feelings about it all right, but they are choosing to ignore them by trying to pretend that they don't exist. But, they do exist, and pretending won't make them go away.

They need to realize that we all have feelings and have a right to have them be recognized and heard. They are not right or wrong; feelings are. If we felt them, then they exist; they are our feelings. Our feelings are not wrong. We shouldn't try to argue ourselves out of having a right to feel them.

In order to have a chest cold exit the body we need to acquire our soul learning which is to come to resolution with our feelings by recognizing our feelings, and then expressing them to whom or what they are directed at. We must confront the situation in our life right now that we are not expressing our feelings about. If we don't, then all of these feelings of ours will continue to stay bottled up inside of us causing us to continue to have the chest cold.

When energy builds with no place to go a problem is sure to arise. We take energy in not only from seeing, hearing, smelling and touching. All energy in our body must always equally flow in and out.

CIRCULATION

Circulation problems indicate that one's life force – blood - is not flowing throughout the body freely. This condition reflects difficulty with letting things in their life flow freely. Such individuals are having a problem with allowing their life force – their *will* - to be vibrant. They keep things buried deep and hidden within. They are allowing themselves to be hidden and not heard. These people fear life and their place in it. Therefore they are very hesitant about life. They are not aggressive, because life to them is uncertain and their position in life is unclear. Yet this is so only because they are unwilling to discover. They need to learn to be more open-minded in life.

Their soul learning is to let their life freely flow, realizing that there is a place for everybody, and the only way to discover this place is to quit holding themselves back. Rather, they need to put forth action to do something about it. Let go of the rope and dive into life!

COLIC

The basis for colic is that the child is feeling *unsafe* in life. They feel that they're not ready yet to participate in life. This hesitation will be reflected within their body, causing the digestive system to be sluggish and to cramp as it is forced into action when food is taken in. The child is having trouble digesting what is going on in their life. As the child wakes up to life, the organs will slowly awaken on their own time. The more the child wakes up to life, accepting life, the more the particular organs will kick into action. The parents or caregivers should provide the child with *safety*, letting the child know that they are there, that it is time to wake up and that it is safe to do so.

When the child is going through this process they are really bothered, and it is best to try and make them feel as comfortable as we can. Eventually, this troublesome time will pass as the child becomes more secure and decides to open up to life. Such children only remain closedbecause they don't know what to expect. They fear life until they gain the soul learning and feel *secure*. This is why it is important for the caregiver to provide *security*. If the caregiver is nervous, the child will sense this nervousness, which only reinforces their uncertainty. Therefore, it is important to remain calm. The *big key* for this soul through this process is to provide them with as much security as possible.

COLON

The biggest issue for those who acquire colon problems is that they don't feel that they deserve anything. They feel that they have fallen by the wayside and so their colon therefore behaves accordingly. These individuals are ultimately unhappy with who they have become. They have not achieved what they would have liked to, in their terms.

The soul learning for these individuals is to believe in themselves and realize that the main reason that they have not achieved their dreams is because they have lacked the self-confidence to believe in themselves enough to do it.

COLITIS

Those who acquire colitis are at a time in their life where they wonder where they are going and what their place is in life. They are trying too hard to keep up with the rate that things are coming at them. Too much is going on, more than they are able to deal with. Things are happening too quickly. They don't know what could possibly be coming next for them. They question, *"Can I go on?"*

The cramping of colitis signifies the constrictive and restrictive motion of indecision from *"Yes, I can go on,"* to *"No, I can't go on"*. These individuals need to relax, slow down and realize that indeed they can go on, and will go on. God never gives us more than we are capable of handling. Though, we may not know where things are heading, we must remember that there is always a divine plan in store for all of us.

COMA

An individual in a coma is lost in the realm of possibilities within their brain. They have no knowledge or recognition of the conscious state of "here" and "now." It is similar to a catatonic state, yet these individuals are not frozen in their mind as a catatonic individual is. Rather they are traveling about very freely in the realm of possibilities within their mind. When the coma occurred the individual dived into their mind, going deep into the realm of possibilities. When there, they get caught up in these possibilities and lost touch with this reality – life. Once there, it is difficult to find the path back.

A key factor in finding the pathway back into this conscious state is whether the individual has a strong drive or will for life – a purpose that is urging them to come back. If they think and feel there is no real importance or purpose to come back for, then it's easier for them to lose touch with this life. They begin to loose their identity, the purpose and reason for existence, and soon there seems to be no need to find their way back.

These individuals are *lost*, yet they don't even realize that they are lost. Many times, their consciousness will lead them back once it feels that it has something still left to do here. Therefore, it tries to lead the individual (whole consciousness) back. Yet, if the individual resists coming back to this level of consciousness because they don't feel and think that there is a purpose or reason, then they cannot come back. They have given up. Giving up is truly the only reason we die from dis-ease. We give up at one or all levels/states of consciousness. When someone is in a coma, they will stay there until one day they decide: either to come back, with a purpose, or to give up and die.

What can caregivers and loved ones do on this end? First understand that the patient does hear one, so try to stimulate the individual to lead them back. Try to communicate to them, letting them know there are many reason for them to want to stay. Let them know that there is much left for them to do. Or, if you know there were things they wanted to do but felt that they weren't possible, express to them just how possible they can be.

The soul learning for individuals who experience coma is that while they are traveling about in their realm of possibilities, they need to find an avenue or way to come back and put some of the possibilities that exist for their soul into application. They lost connection with the factual world, the conscious state, so that they would have to open up to look at some possibilities that they had been unwilling to consider before.

CONGESTION
(SEE ALSO CHEST COLDS)

Congestion comes about because there is too much energy coming in and not enough going out. This whole process came about because the individual is undergoing an experience where they are not able to understand either the circumstances or the outcome. Because they cannot understand the outcome, they are having a hard time coming to terms with it. They are experiencing a conflict of ideas. They are running away with ideas, but unable to come to any conclusion. There is a *lost sense of direction.*

They are feeling left out, as if they don't have a place because a place was not made for them. The energy is building within, and over time without a conclusion it becomes congested energy, because there is no place for it to go. This is no place for it to go. Congestion in the chest (chest cold) is related to feelings that have no outlet, while congestion in the head (head cold) reflects thoughts that have not been put into action. Thoughts and feelings are pouring in or welling up with no place to go. Because the person does not know what to do with the excess energy, it becomes congested.

Their soul learning is that they need to identify the thoughts and feelings that are building, and work through them rather than just letting them build. They need to try to find understanding and placement for an outlet of the overload. Not until they do will the congestion clear up. They need a new positive outlook on the source of the disturbance, whether it is within themselves, their career, a relationship or some other aspect of their life.

CONJUCTIVITIES

While conjunctivitis, commonly known as *pink eye* the eye gets pink and blood shot. This is due from one over straining to see something in their life right now. They have over viewed a situation in their life too long, trying to force themselves to see it. They are having a difficult time being able to see their capabilities in the current situation.

The itching that often accompanies this dis-ease is a signification of how irritated one is at what they are seeing, looking at in their life right now. They are viewing things too factual; looking only at the tangible and not what is possible. They are stuck because they cannot see anything else as possible in their current situation. Their soul learning is to be open to possibilities about the current situation; seeing the old things in a new light and in different ways.

CONSTIPATION

Individuals with constipation have developed a certain mindset that has caused them to slow down all over. When we mentally start to slow down and don't *perform*, the body follows. Overall, they have slowed down and have become too hesitant when it comes to participating in life, because they think that they are no longer good enough. They question whether they are capable, so they stop doing. They slow down, thus the body slows down, that is, it gets constipated. The systems no longer run smoothly and efficiently.

Because they fear they are not capable, they often don't attempt things in life because they don't want to fail. Their soul learning, what is to go beyond the fear of questioning their capabilities, and worrying about failure, so that they can again begin to engage in life. By doing this, they will then see that they are indeed capable and good enough. This will spark the systems in the body to re-engage, and the body will regain its fluidity.

CONVULSIONS

Individuals who have convulsions have a sudden change in brain waves. When an excessive amount of energy is focused or forced in one direction, the brain over-loaded and loses its original focus, its original brain wave pattern. It jumps off track, so to speak. Taking the normal brain state to its limit causes an overload, in this case resulting in convulsions. The convulsions usually help put the brain back on track, releasing the built-up pressure through the muscular activity of the convulsion itself.

Individuals who are prone to convulsions have a particular personality type. They are commonly the ones that have to prove things to themselves. They are always doing many things to prove *I can, I can*. They take on a lot of duties to try to make up for this insecurity, this sense that they are missing something within. What they need to realize is that they can never fulfill their inner needs with external things. They must feel this security within. They must feel secure within themselves, instead to proving themselves externally.

They tend to go on extensive binges, focusing all of their energy to the point of exhaustion on doing something to prove a point. They jump from one area to another, trying to find the perfect thing that makes them feel better. When the individual gets so focused and the body is being made to overperform so harshly, it loses its focus and jumps from one thing to the next. The brain does the same when pushed to extremes: it switches brain waves, thus inducing a convulsion.

Their soul learning is to become more relaxed in life, letting things flow freely as they come. They need to learn to open up to other possibilities in life, instead of focusing all of their energy in one direction. When they learn to be a little more versatile in their approach to life, and stop forcing the body to prove itself, the body no longer needs to convulse in order to get back on track again. This will help them to learn that true security comes from within.

COUGHS

An individual who coughs is unable to express himself or herself clearly. They have a lot of congested emotional energy because their true feelings are locked and stored within, unable to be expressed and have an outlet. The cough represents the built-up energy coming out.

The individual feels unable to express who they truly are. There is a conflict between who they are and who they think they should be. They feel unable to express who they are inside, so what actually does get expressed on the outside doesn't match what's inside. The conflict creates an emotional upheaval, which leads to the coughing.

Their soul learning is that they need to find a way, avenue or means to express themselves and stop questioning whether it's possible. They need to start expressing and being - who they are.

CROHN'S DISEASE

Crohn's dis-ease develops from an individual who as trouble with their self-identity. They question "who they really are" and "where they are really headed in life. "When some circumstance or situation arises in their life that brings about this question, the abdomen will become inflamed and symptoms will increase. The self is lost and at conflict. These individuals face inflammation because ultimately they are inflamed; upset or bothered about themselves at the time.

Their soul learning is that they need to learn to love and accept themselves for who they are and where they are at in life. If they continue to be upset or hold on to resentment over it, they face further difficulty. They must stop trying to push themselves to be more, often by doing more. They need to let life flow naturally for them and then all things will come in the right divine time. Pushing it is not going to get one where they want to be any quicker.

Learn to be happy with who they are and where they are at in life. If we let life lead us where we need to go, it will happen, but not by forcing it, only by accepting what is; who we are and where we are at now, letting the rest fall into place. It will, if we let it. It is the forcing that causes the conflict and ultimately the inflammation by trying to make ourselves more capable than we are at the present time. Just like the diarrhea that accompanies this dis-ease comes from the individual trying to take on too much at one time. They are simply not capable to handle all that is going on.

D

DEPRESSION

Individuals who face depression are dealing with a great inner despair. They have lost their place in life. They question, "How can I go on in life *feeling this way?*" Often they have just been through one or more traumatic emotional experiences that have left them feeling lost and hopeless about how to go on, how to go forward in life. They are stuck in grief. This grief has left them feeling hopeless. Depression can easily lead to suicide, depending on the degree of the depression. They need to find a way to remember that there is a sunnier side of life. Right now they are stuck in a dark cloud. They need to regain hope that there is a way forward.

The soul learning of depression is that they must come to understand that all things that occur are divine and are only meant to bring each of us to the next stage of life for our soul's growth. They need to begin to trust that there is always hope, to search for it and hang on to it. Hope gives the power, strength and peace to overcome whatever life sends. *Hope* is the only thing that will lift this feeling of such despair.

DIABETES

This dis-ease comes to individuals who cannot totally face or handle situations as they are. They are unable to take things as they come, so they are often unhappy with life. They always want the situation to change, but only the way they think it should change. If they can't have things as they wish, they will often be stubborn to the point where they will hold back. They are ultimately only hurting themselves by denying themselves, because of needing to have everything their way.

These individual's soul learning is to accept what life has brought their way. They need to release their control, to stop trying to change things in and accept things and people, including them self, as they are. When they learn to enjoy what is, than happiness and joy can flow freely abundantly again.

DIARRHEA

Diarrhea occurs when an individual is dealing with an overload. Their underlying issue is questioning whether they are *capable* of mastering a certain situation that they are facing. They don't think they have what it takes.

These individuals are judging themselves too harshly and spending too much time an analyzing the matter at hand. They do this because they think and feel inadequate. Therefore, because they are trying to make up for their self-diagnosed inadequacy, they push things along too fast, faster than they are truly capable of handling at this time. Thus, their body cannot process all of this energy enough quickly, so literally it goes right through them, leading to diarrhea.

The soul learning for these individuals is that they need to slow down, stop trying to out-do themselves and let the process of life run freely at its own pace. They need to learn not to force themselves more than they are capable of handling.

DISC PROBLEMS
(SEE BACK PROBLEMS)

Disc problems appear when an individual who is putting an enormous amount of pressure on them selves, either in general or in a specific circumstance in their life. This pressure is a very scattered energy. In other words, the individual is putting excessive pressure on himself or herself to perform, without really knowing if all of it is necessary. They think if it as a full-proof method of covering all territories.

Their soul learning is to evaluate what they currently pouring too much energy into. They need to determine what is important and then learn to let the unnecessary go. They need to find a direction for their excessive energy, rather than just burning themselves out. Then the energy in theirr body will begin to flow in harmony again.

DIGESTIVE PROBLEMS

Individuals who have digestive problems are having a hard time accepting the circumstances or situations in their life. They are literally having trouble digesting them. Things are coming at them too quickly, quicker than they're able to digest, which is the underlying problem. They don't just question whether they *can* go on; they question whether they *want* to go on. They are very uncertain about their place and direction in life; they can't see it at this time.

Their soul learning is that they need to accept that the life experiences that come their way are exactly divine, although they may not see it as divine or understand its meaning at the time. They need to learn to accept things in life freely as they are, knowing that it is for the overall good of their well-being.

DRUG ADDICTION

These individuals are trapped by their own insecurity and doubt. The fix for this dis-ease is *self- confidence*, so that they can find themselves and a place for themselves in life. his is their true search. They feel that life that has no possible place for them. Because they feel that so they run to an alternative: a hiding place deep within which they reach through drugs.

They question their ability. They feel that they are not capable of *being* or *becoming* anything in life. This is what gives them a low self-esteem. They don't like who they are, although they will try to convince you differently because they are fighting to save the little identity that is left.

Because they are not capable of being where they think they should be, they often don't participate where they are. They end up refraining from life. They avoid becoming aggressive and end up allowing life and the opportunities in it to pass them by. Often they blame and punish others for not going, doing, becoming, having, when really the root cause is *back at the self and nobody else.*

Ultimately, they are having trouble accepting who they are and where they're at, and only they can do something about it. Even though they are scared and question their capability, they need to keep in mind that we all question our abilities at some time in our lives, yet we must all still participate in life. These individuals need to "invest" themselves in something they desire to become, instead of running and hiding. Sure, it is hard, and requires much effort, but the reward is miraculous.

These individuals need help to learn how to acquire coping skills, that is, on how to handle things without running or hiding from them. They need guidance to help them find a life for them self, to learn how to let themselves come out of the box and not hide within or cover themselves up. They need to just let themselves *be* who they are and know that it is OK – that it's safe.

These individuals soul learning is to accept themselves and things for what they are, and then find a goal and go after it. Their motto must become "you can do It!" These individuals need to turn into fighters, not outside of themselves, where they fight too much already, but rather fighters within. They need to build *self-confidence* and then come out fighting like a tiger.

E

EARACHES

Individuals who develop an earache are those who are having a hard time taking in any more information on a given subject. They are stuck in a situation and cannot see a promising outlook for themselves. It seems as if they don't want to hear any more, because they don't. Now they are avoiding even hearing about it or facing it in any way. The ear has become blocked up because they are blocked, or in other words they are being *closed-minded* about it. They are not open to hear any more possibilities, because they have heard too many of the facts, and, based on that, things look dim.

Their soul learning is to *be open* to new ideas and ways to go about this certain subject, as well as with other things in life. They need to look at is *what can be* if they allow themselves to open up and stop avoiding it.

These individuals need to take some time to be open and aware to the universe for guidance about the situation in their life. The soul sends messages in a multitude of ways, such as from others around us, a radio, a billboard, a sign, etc. They must learn to give their soul some time and it will guide and show them the way. But, in order to see or hear what our soul is telling us, you will have to be *open* and willing to accept what is being told to us.

EDEMA

Fluid retention comes about because fluid stays stored in one place and builds, rather than freely flowing throughout the body. The fluid becomes congested energy, which gets lodged into certain areas and is unable to flow freely, because the individual is unable to allow them selves to flow freely in life. They are unable to adapt to the current circumstances in their life. In the case of edema in the feet, our feet metaphorically represent our walk in life. Therefore, edema of the feet signifies that one is not freely taking the steps that need to be takes, which would allow energy to freely flow instead of pooling in one place.

This stagnation or pooling occurs because the individual experiencing a *loss of a clear direction.* They are carrying a deep sense of not being able to understand what they should be doing about a certain situation or circumstance that is currently going on, or in their life overall. The scope of the learning is reflected in whether they live with this condition all the time or whether just has just recently come about.

Because this individual does not have a clear-cut pattern to work with in their life, the body does not have a plan to work with either. This means that the fluid does not know where to go, what to do. This is why the body is making so much fluid: they have too many ideas, too many possible steps that could be taken, that they don't end up taking because they fear it to be the wrong step. In other words, the "steps untaken" are causing the feet and ankles to swell. This fluid or energy will build up until they pick a direction that they believe is the right direction no matter what anybody says or thinks - and go with it. They need to quit worrying about it being the right direction or about whatever others say is the right direction: Just pick one and stick to it. This will allow the body to release the fluid. The overall soul learning is this: pick a direction, a plan of action, and run with it. Don't waste any more time.

EMPHYSEMA

Individuals who develop emphysema have for a long time been living a lifestyle where they have kept in their feelings about many things and tried to pretend that everything is OK. The problem is that everything is really *not OK*. They have too many hurts that they have let stay hidden for too long. They have an inner need to make everything ok, not just with themselves, but with others as well. They don't like to create waves, feeling that they have caused trouble or hurt by expressing their feelings. They will hold their true feelings in, even though they are terribly distressed within, just to keep the peace.

The soul learning for these individuals soul learning is to learn to confront the situation or person when their feelings are not OK. They need to express their feelings, release them. By keeping feelings in, they are literally smothering themselves out of life. This pattern of pretending that everything is OK has been there a long time. Therefore, this soul learning process is going to take some time.

As with any dis-ease, when one learns this soul learning and then puts it into application emphysema can be overcome. The more completely one learns the more the emphysema will improve. The next generation benefits too, because both "finished" and "unfinished" soul learnings are passed on to children, so that they can continue the learning. This is how the soul evolves and grows. Some learnings can take a short time, others lifetimes. How hard it is to acquire a soul learning depends on how much growth a person's ancestors have had in this particular learning as well as the growth the person is able to gain in his or her lifetime.

ENDOMETRIOSIS

Endometriosis is a dis-ease process related to an expression of ones femininity changing and evolving. It's sometimes called *the career girls disease.* A women with endometriosis has a conflict with not being able to fulfill her inborn desire to nurture, as well to have a career or position outside of the home, thus changing her role for what it means to be a woman now in life: her feminine role.

Opposing this process growth and wanting to stay with known styles of feminine expression only causes greater problems. Having a mindset that mothers should stay home, that femininity has no peace outside of the home is opposed to the newly forming mindset. This internal conflict begins to affect the body, particularly the female organs. Blame and guilt are the destructive forces that eat away at women with this dis-ease:guilt for not feeling completely perfect at being able to balance both aspects of them selves as a woman.

The woman's female organs are trying to adapt, yet because she is having difficulty with this adjustment, endometriosis forms: the endometriosis tissue is *out of place*. The endometriosis tissue is out of place because she is trying to find a new place for herself. This is a newly discovered avenue of self-expression of her femininity. If the woman accepts the new expression of her femininity, rather than opposing it by hanging on to the old mindset, then her body will adapt more easily. However, she may have difficulty figuring out how to deal with this new form of her feminine expression As a result, her body will have difficulty adapting to this new process and so she will experience the discomfort of endometriosis.

To help this endometriosis tissue, she must find new ways to cope with her new change in being as a woman. Women must learn new forms of feminine expression of themselves that works for their current position in life. For each woman this expression will be different. The learning for many women today is to achieve this task of new female expression. It may take few or many experiences to acquire this learning; the learning may need to be passed down to the next generation for further learning. Until the learning is understood, it will continue to be passed down through the generations.

Whenever she feels that she has not been able to accomplish this balance, she feels imperfect. When she feels imperfect in any way then she becomes unhappy with herself, as well as any form of creative expression that comes from her. She spends a great deal of time trying to cover up for these imperfections that she sees in herself.

The soul learning for these individuals is that they need to realize that it is not about being perfect or having it *right*, it just about being the best that we can be with the circumstance presented to us. These individuals need to learn to love themselves and be happy for who they are, and what we are, having being given the opportunity to accomplish what they have.

EPILESPSY

Epilepsy is characterized by seizures that are induced by electrical impulses in the brain that cause the brain to cease, in an attempt to get itself back on track. It is like shaking somebody to get them out of a state of shock, yet the brain does this to itself, to wake itself up before it closes off.

Those who carry this condition are individuals who tend to run from things that they don't want to deal with. They are avoiding the obvious, so the brain must cease on occasion in order to wake itself up. These individuals are choosing to not notice things that are needed. Therefore, their souls need to be forced to look at things, to stop hiding from them and choosing to ignore them.

They need to learn to face experiences by stating their own truths: their thoughts, feelings and beliefs.

When we don't state our truth, we are denying ourselves: we close a part of ourselves down, thus closing our ability to grow and expand. Over time, we become closed and resentful. Therefore, it is vital to openly express who we are and to remain open to what life brings our way.

The reason these individuals avoid dealing with things is that they haven't yet learned *how* to deal with them. Yet, the only way for them to learn how is to face the experience and cope through it. These individuals see things as impossible. They don't see a fix. In their eyes, it is impossible because they are not open to new ways to deal with the situation. They are too stuck with rigid patterns of how things were and how they used to deal with them. Their soul learning is to step into the world of possibilities, to be open to the new and to look at themselves and life in a new light.

EPSTEIN BARR VIRUS

This virus causes an *overreaction* by the immune system, which eventually leads to a *burnout* of the immune system. Someone who suffers the effects of this virus goes through a severe depression that doesn't match is the text book diagnosis. This is because this virus attacks *all the states* of our being, as a whole: mentally, (thoughts), emotionally, (feelings), spiritually, (beliefs) and physically, (behaviors), all at once – like a big burnout. In other words, they have gotten to a point in their life where they have tried to *play the game* so long, that it is now catching up with them. They have burned them selves out at all levels.

These individuals have a very hard time accepting that they need to be cared for. They conveniently avoid getting their needs met. They don't allow the circumstances to arise to get their needs meet. They are not consciously aware of the extent to which they avoid this **love** that they need. Instead they try to provide it to themselves, or try to make up for it in other ways. They do this as a defense mechanism, keeping others at a safe distance, due to their fear of rejection. *"Rejection of what?"*Love!Since they experienced rejection a long time ago, they have blocked any risk of feeling it again. They have also interpreted many other situations as being rejected. Therefore, they have spent much energy and time blocking themselves from any further rejections.

They fear that they won't actually get what they need, so they avoid it all together. That way, there's no letdown.

Their soul learning is that *no man is an island alone.* These individuals need to let themselves open up, even though they fear it. We all fear it, but it's all part of life.

These individuals stopped receiving help and love from others because they feared rejection. They don't speak up for their needs because they are afraid that they will be turned down, due to past rejection, so they won't go there. They won't be vulnerable, so they don't put themselves in positions where their needs can be met. But they need to learn that if they don't allow themselves to be vulnerable, then their needs will *never* be met. They need to overcome the rejection that they have felt in the past. Even though they fear the hurt, they need to put themselves in those situations and learn to trust again. This is the only way to overcome the virus and its effects.

The objective of this virus is to put them in a position were they must care for themselves. Eventually, they must learn to allow themselves to be open and accept *in* love and care from others. With that love and care, they will realize that they really had nothing to fear in the first place, that there was a safe environment wanting to provide for them all along.

EYES – FARSIGHTED

These individuals have difficulty seeing things up close. They are farsighted because they keep their sights on the future. Kept in balance, this is a good trait but in this case it's too much. It has become rather became the predominant way through which they are viewing the world – from afar.

They are our daydreamers: open to the possibilities in life, yet closed to the facts before them. They are unable to see things up close because they avoid looking at what's right in front of them their life, often because it's tuough and they don't want to face it.

The soul learning is that they need to learn to pay more attention to the facts in front of them. The more they begin to pay attention to look at the situations right in front of them and deal with them, thus accepting them for what they are, the more their ability to see physiologically will alter as well. Eventually, they will wake up to see what is passing them by.

EYES – NEARSIGHTED

These individuals have difficulty seeing things far away. They are nearsighted because they have trouble seeing the future in their life. They have a hard time seeing what will be because they are closed to possibilities. They see little as possible in life for themselves. They are stuck in the now and won't allow themselves to go forward into the future because they don't want to face the future.

The soul learning for these individuals is that although we currently do not know what the future will hold, all is gracefully divine. Even if the past has shown us unpleasant experiences, we must realize that the reason was for the greater whole of our life. These unpleasant experiences helped us to understand many things in life. These experiences have made us stronger in many ways. We need to look at these experiences for our learning. They are only present to help us grow, learn and gain more from life. There is much potential waiting to be discovered in the future.

F

FATIGUE

General fatigue is often brought on when an individual is at a point in their life where he has lost some of their gusto. Contrary to what you might think, it's not because they have over done things and gotten tired out. Rather, they are tired on the outside because they are tired inside. They are giving up their fight. They are not standing up for *who they are* and their position in life. This happens because one is questioning their worth, and whether they really have a position or place in life.

Fatigue occurs when a person is extending them self and not getting enough back out of it. It is not just a matter of doing too much. As long as we are getting a return for our effort, we can do a lot, in fact all we want. The problem is when we think there's a mismatch between what we're getting out and what we are putting in. All levels are involved: physically, mentally, emotionally and spiritually. It boils down to what we give ourselves. For example, even if we are not receiving recognition from others, as long as we feel it so within, then that is all that counts.

If we are giving ourselves back what we are giving out, we will be OK, even if nobody around us is giving us anything for our efforts. Most of this satisfaction comes from within, so if we can supply it for ourselves, then we can give all we want. This is why it is so important that we feel happy about what we are doing in life. If we are not, then we are not going to give our body the energy it needs to continue. The thrill will vanish, and we are sure to be tired over the simplest things.

The problem for individuals suffering from fatigue is that they have given out so much that they are now giving up. They must not let themselves give up. This only makes things worse for their body and their life. Rather, they need to spark that flame within – ignite it!If they are not happy with themselves and what they are doing in their life, than they are not going to feed themselves back that thrill, the inner fulfillment they need. If that flame is gone, then they need a new direction. This could be a minor or major shift, either within the realm of what they are currently doing or on a whole new path. In either case, their soul learning is to do something that does provide them with internal desire and happiness, which is the fuel for their flame of energy. Then they will have energy, because they will now again be inspired!

FEARS

Fears are those things in our lives that we desperately try to avoid, so that we do not have to face them. The reason we don't want to face them is that they lead our mind back to the negative experience that we faced to begin with that turned into the fear.

We learn a fear through an unpleasant experience. The more impact the experience had on us the greater the fear becomes. From that negative experience we retain a certain memory that holds the way that our mind was able to deal with the experience at the time. The way that we were able to understand it was based on our interpretation of it at the time, which is unique to each individual.

When we start to interpret a situation, before it becomes a fear, we analyze it along with the facts and experiences that we have in relation to the situation. When we do this we are looking for an answer. An answer is a type of mental explanation that allows us to put the experience to rest. By putting it to rest, or, in other words, coming to terms with it, we learn to understand it. Sometimes we don't have all the knowledge necessary to make an analysis, so we can't put the experience to rest. Instead, we carry these unsettled emotions with no placement for them within us. Over time, if we are not able to gain this knowledge, then those emotions become fears. And fears they remain until we learn how to come to terms with these negative emotions by trying to face them before they reach the stage of dis-ease. It is not until we learn how to come to terms with a situation, by being able to understand the soul learning it carries, that we are then able to put it to rest.

The severity of the fear depends on the degree to which we were unable to analyze, come to terms with and put to rest the experience we encountered. If it was not possible to deal with the experience at all, then re-encountering a similar situation can induce a catatonic state. From there the level of intensity decreases.

Fears are glitches that we carry with us for life until we face them. We need to willingly pull our fears to us, because ultimately we do anyway. First, we have to acquire the additional knowledge we need in order to analyze the initial experience and put it to rest. We gain this knowledge by going through other relational experiences that give us the opportunity to better understand this fear/learning. Once we have this knowledge, we are then better equipped to analyze the experience. At that point, we will pull the fear back to us so that we can face it again, to overcome it. When we now live it, since we have a greater understanding from our new experiences, now having gained more knowledge, we will look at it differently and thus interpret it differently. It will no longer be a fear because we now have come to understand it. So, a fear is really a misinterpretation of an experience, due to a lack of knowledge.

Fears are our soul learnings. We must learn to not avoid our fears when presented with the opportunity to face them head on, even though our distress may be intense. We need to look at what we fear in different ways so that we can learn to understand it. We need to escape being stuck on what the past has told us. By re-facing the experience and seeking the positive in it, we can then regain a feeling of safety.

Fears can be "blocks to becoming". Avoiding our fears, which we ultimately must face anyway, only stops us from having the opportunities our soul needs to further grow. Overall, we have to move beyond our fears or we will get stuck, block ourselves from further growth, and usually end up with dis-ease as a last attempt for our soul learning.

FEVER

One who acquires a fever is burning up inside over a negative experience, and is now trying to burn some of it off. These individuals are upset or bothered about something so much that their emotions are boiling over. They have a one-track mind about something: that they have thought about it over and over again and can see no way to fix or solve it. They act much more calm, cool and collected on the outside than they really are in the inside. They pretend everything is OK, but it's not. In fact, not at all!

A fever is a way that the body can naturally, literally, let off some steam so a person can calm down and maybe look at the inside in a more levelheaded way. There is something going on that they don't see a fix for. They ask, "How is it ever going to happen?" Yet, they don't just think about it and ponder over it; they actually let it affect them emotionally as well. They are just plain pissed off that they can't see a way out.

So they do need to calm down, cool off and be open to taking a different approach to the situation, rather than looking at it the same old stubborn way. They need to broaden their horizons and get out of the box. They need to let the universe show them the way.

FOOD POISIONING

Food poisoning strikes an individual when they are ready to give up: to call it quits on something's existence a job, a relationship, life itself. They are unable to deal with the way things are any longer. They have been trying to "hold the fort" for too long, and they can't handle the stress and expectations any longer. Food poisoning is a clear sign that a person rejects their present situation.

An individual who acquires food poisoning needs to take a look at their life and evaluate why their body is showing signs of rejection. Their soul learning is to identify the situation that is poisonous to them and expel the crisis from their life. They aren't able to continue to live with it any longer, because it is truly poison to them. They need, somewhere in their life, to find a new start, a new direction.

G

GALL BLADDER

Individuals who develop gall bladder problems have for a long time, been having a hard time digesting what life has brought to them. They now wonder if they even want to go on. They have purposely avoided dealing with situations for so long, and created a big storage house of backed up energy from things they haven't dealt with. Now that back up of energy is eating away at them, thus affecting the gall bladder.

Their soul learning is that they need to let go of some of the things in the past that didn't turn out favorably in their eyes. Instead they can begin to see that everything is divine and necessary at the time. They need to come to terms with the old and let go of it in order to move on in the present. They need to accept and take on the new things that come their way, saying to themselves *I do want to go on*, or things will only get worse.

GLAUCOMA

Those who develop glaucoma are individuals who are lost. They can't really see where they are going in life. They are stuck in the present situation, with no visible way out in their eyes. They can't see what the future holds for them or where it is going, so they start avoiding even looking at the future, and therefore the dis-ease process that creates glaucoma begins.

These individuals see limited possibilities for themselves in the future. Therefore a limited perception of their life based on certain facts as they see them. They think of themselves as realists, only seeing the tangible and avoiding the vast possibilities in their life. By not bothering to look any further into the opportunities in life, they will soon lose the ability to *see* life at all.

The soul learning for these individuals is that if they want to eliminate this dis-ease they must change their outlook and become more open-minded individuals. They must not give up hope. Once they give up hope and the dis-ese is inevitable at the physical level, the dis-ease becomes the learning. Now that their ability to see has been removed, this loss will make them learn to look deeper into life for other ways to learn. They will have to become more aware and sensitive of what's up ahead for them, instead of avoiding it.

GOUT

Gout is a condition deriving from the presence of too much uric acid in the body, which that leads to crystallization in the bones causing pain and stiffness. Individuals who have gout are too responsive to things in life. They also tend to be too *opinionated*. They have something to say about everything. They are compelled to be on top of things. They feel if they miss something, then they may be left behind. In fear of being left behind, they always involve themselves in everything they can find. With these individuals, it is not just that they must be involved with things, but rather they must be *on top of things*. They feel that gives them an edge, so they can be a step above everybody else. This is the only way they truly feel comfortable. This is their safety zone because of their true insecurity. Yet, these over-responsive actions lead to an over-production of uric acid in the joints and bones. The stiffness of gout keeps them from being able to *over-respond*. Now, through this dis-ease they are put in a situation where they can't respond. Rather, they have to contemplate and realize that they do not have to be on top to be important.

Their learning results from not having a clear path in their life. They are always going and doing, having many avenues, yet they do not have a clear or definite path to follow in life. These people need a position or status in life. This is why they have to be on top of things, because they want to appear as if they have a hole. They are seeking *prestige*.

The soul learning for these individuals soul learning is to realize that true *prestige* comes from within, the honor we give ourselves in whatever we do. They need to take time to search for the path in life that is right for them, not basing their choice on the external world of standards for prestige. True stature comes from within and can only be known by one self. Life is truly not about being *on top;* rather, it's about being who you are and giving who you are, and then the true prestige within in you unfolds.

GUM PROBLEMS

Individuals facing problems with their gums have been letting something eat away at them for too long. In other words, they have japed their jaws too much (talked too much) about the subject. These individuals in general talk too much about everything, rather than just being and expressing their true selves, without having to outdo themselves.

Because they talk they are not getting a chance to get their true needs met. Their true needs aren't getting a chance even to be expressed, let alone heard. Such people are too busy expressing trivial stuff, rather than what's really important. They're too busy trying to get more, when that's not what really makes them happy. The soul leaning is that they need to learn to listen more and express more of the important things in their life, instead of staying stuck expressing the trivial things over and over again.

H

HEAD COLDS
(SEE ALSO COLDS)

Head colds arise when someone has an enormous amount of congested mental energy. Such individuals have too many thoughts about a particular issue without having any understanding of them. They cannot see a fix or a fit. They have thought through something to the point where all the facts are laid before them, and they still cannot see how they or it is going to happen, work. They've thought about it to the point that they are sick over it.

Their problem is that they have looked at too many facts. They have analyzed and intellectualized too much. Their soul learning is to become more opened-minded by looking at new possibilities and ways to solve their problems, rather than continuing to go about it the same way, to the point of getting sick over it.

They need to let their feelings in on this one. Rather than trying to think it out to come up with a solution, they need to "feel" their way through to the solution. They should experiment with letting their feelings guide them, even if the path of what those feelings suggest doesn't fully make sense at the time. Over time, the right way will show itself.

HEADACHES

Headaches occur when individuals are under stress in a current situation. They are stressed out because they can't figure out what to do. They don't have the answers they need to be at ease within themselves.

Yet, they keep searching for this understanding. These individuals won't just put things to rest within their mind. Rather, the search consumes them. Thoughts circulate around and around within their minds until the energy builds to a boiling point and as a result a headache emerges. Headaches represent excessive mental energy: thinking too much with no placement or understanding for our thoughts.

We can think all we want without any trouble as long as we have placement (an understanding gained from past experience) for our thoughts. This kind of thinking keeps things perpetuating and energy flowing. The problem arises when we get stuck with our thinking. When we can't see a fit for something and how it is going to work and so forth. We can't come to a conclusion let our mind come to rest, so it keeps going. This energy builds and gets stuck, causing a headache.

People prone to headaches get stuck because, based on their facts, they can't see things working out. The problem is that they keep trying to use the same old solutions and it is, just not working, so they are stuck. They are too fact-orientated. They need to learn to open themselves up to new ideas and ways of looking at themselves or the situation at hand.

People who get headaches frequently have a need to *see* how things work. The more intense the headaches are, the more the person has tried to over force themself to *see* and understand something. The soul learning needed for these individuals is to be more open-minded, to have more creative thinking and less constructive thinking. They need to think *outside of the box*.

HEARING PROBLEMS

Individuals who develop hearing problems are starting to shut down their sensory channels to the outside world. They get caught up in their own world, so they tend to shut off what's going on around them. They are too busy listening inward by, just themselves, instead of learning to listen to others around them. Learning to listen to what others are telling them can help them have a better understanding in the world outside.

Their soul learning is they need to discipline themselves to not have selective hearing, taking in only what they want to hear, but to take in as what they need to hear, what those around them are expressing to them. Because they don't want to listen to what others have to say, being so caught up in their own needs, they often end up with little to no learning. They need to be better listeners so that they can take in the beauty and the vast possibilities in life by learning to listen to others, even at times when they don't really want to. They will learn a lot more about life and what's going on around them by learning to listen to what others have to say. This will make them more knowledgeable about life and the things and people in life beside just themselves.

If this learning is not acquired they could end up sealed permanently, in their own silent world. This isolation would be the result of avoiding the outside world and choosing to live mainly in their own world, forgetting about others and life around them. Over time, if the individual does not learn this soul learning, they will lose all sense of the world of sound around them, hearing only what's inside them.

HEART ATTACK

A heart attack results when one experiences an overload of emotions that have been built up for a long time and are now bursting through *at the seams*.

A recent circumstance or situation was the final trigger to set off the heart attack - the straw that broke the camel's back, so to speak. This event triggered a particular feeling that had been bothering the person for a long time and had built up. This last situation was another reminder of this particular feeling, which became the overload that set off the attack.

The soul learning for such individuals is to learn to work with their emotions freely:in other words, learning to express their feelings freely as they arise as appropriate to the circumstance or situation. They must learn to not let these emotions go unsettled. These individuals need to learn to express their feelings per situation, instead of letting them build until they're ready to burst.

These individuals think they have things under control, when really there is an emotion that they need to confront. They get themselves involved in too many things in life by taking on too much. They want to be able to change things, to make them be OK for everybody. They must come to see that they can't take care of it all. Certain things are out of their hands so they need to let go.

HEARTBURN

Individuals who have heartburn cannot just let everything be OK – let things come to a rest. They feel everything deep within and that bothers them. They cannot let it go. This feeling may be about a certain situation that just occurred, or they may just be this type of personality. This distinction determines whether they have heartburn occasionally or frequently.

They harbor their feelings about things, and eventually these feelings turn bitter and begin the dis-ease process that results is heartburn: They develop a backup of old stored emotions that have become bitter and need a way out. Since the individual is not able to deal with them by putting them to rest, dwelling on them stirs up further bitterness.

Their soul learning is to learn to let things be, instead of harboring the situation. They need to learn to deal with it and accept it for what it is, learn from it and move on, and then the heartburn will be alleviated.

HEMORRHOIDS

Hemorrhoids are due to an individual straining or forcing themselves to do something. This effort could be physical, mental, emotional or spiritual. In other words, if it's one's nature to be too responsive the result will probably be hemorrhoids. The individual is over-doing in order to prove them self.

Instead of spending so much time trying to force things, they should rather be looking at why they have to use force in the first place. There is an area in their life physically, mentally, emotionally or spiritually where they are trying to force something. This area needs to be evaluated, because we should not have to force something to be; it should pass freely if it's meant to be. Their soul learning is to learn not to force things to be, but rather to let them bloom on their own.

HEPATITIS

Hepatitis occurs in those individuals who are out to prove a point, to make known their anger and retribution. This reaction arises from the deep hurt and suffering that they are encountering at the time the dis-ease occurs. Those who contract this virus have pulled it to themselves like a magnet in order to surface some long-term hurt or anger that is festering within their whole body. This hurt and anger has eaten away at them to the point where the body cannot filter this negative emotion anymore, so it takes over.

These people are the type who cannot just stand back and let things happen as they will. They must put their part in. They have a hard time just accepting things as they come because they want to change things to their liking. They are very picky and bull-headed individuals, liking things a certain way. Nobody is going to show them differently. If they can't have what they want, they will take it out on themselves, often in ways of denying themselves. This causes them harm. They are very tense and particular people, so when upsetting things come up, they cannot just let them go: everything bothers them. Things tend to fester easily. This virus allows them to see how full of anger they are.

Their soul learning is to learn to take all of the energy they are putting into this anger and redirect it into accepting life and allowing love in. They need to learn to turn their strong emotions into love and let go of the anger, by learning to come to terms with their hurt from the past. Life is too short!

HERNIA

Individuals who acquire a hernia have at this point in their life pushed themselves too hard to try to express themselves. They have tried so hard to prove themselves, by trying to be more than they were truly capable of. They have strained their true capabilities and now they are suffering the consequences. They carry an inner desire to prove themselves, a need to stand out in their own eyes. This dis-ease will not allow them to overdo to prove themselves. In fact, this dis-ease will help them learn to accept themselves for who they are and what they really can do.

The soul learning is for them to learn to be happy with who they are, realizing they don't have to do or be more, constantly trying to prove themselves. They don't have a reason to overdo anything. They are perfect just the way they are; what they are capable of.

HIVES

Individuals who develop hives are trying to force something in their life to change because it isn't how they would like it to be. They are very irritated over the way things are. They will not accept that life cannot be the way they wish it to be, so they continue to try to force things to change. An outbreak of hives is an expression of their inner aggravation. Something is really bothering them: it is under their skin, and they can't change it. Because they can't change what is, they feel inadequate so they force things to try to prove differently.

The soul learning for these individuals is to learn to relax and allow themselves to let nature and life take its course, without so much self-involvement. Self-involvement in general is good yes, but it becomes a problem when the self is so involved that it does not leave room for that which needs to happen in one's lives. These individuals have been so busy forcing something that cannot be, that they end up blocking what needs to be.

HODGKINS DIS-EASE

The onset of this dis-ease reflects that the individual is at a stage in their life where they are truly not satisfied with themselves. They are disappointed in what they have become. Their expectations were much higher than they are living up to. In actuality, his or her standards are much too high for almost anybody. These expectations become like an extension ladder with no end. Once they see that they can do more then they will expect more of themselves. For the most part, such people are **very** hard on themselves, causing a lot of undue stress in their lives.

The dis-ease is brought on because of the continued disappointment: their perception that they have disappointed themselves. For the person with Hodgkin's dis-ease, this is an ongoing issue throughout their life: their soul has not been able to live up to their own (unrealistic) standards. Now it has gotten to a point where they are carrying so much self-disappointment that it has built into total *disgust.* They then begin to punish themselves by denying themselves; only this time it's life!

These people are trying to punish themselves: they can't allow themselves to get what they need out of life. They get to a point where they are no longer even willing to try to please themselves, so they just stop altogether and develop a cancerous dis-ease. Individuals who develop this dis-ease do so in attempts to rid themselves of life because they cannot deal with their anguish any longer. But in actuality, they begin to learn about standards and limitations in a different light. Once life is actually at risk, we all look at things in a different manner.

The soul learning that is acquired through this dis-ease is that eventually the person will drive themselves crazy with their unrealistically high expectations and standards. Then they can come to appreciate and honor themselves and where they are at in their life, while they still have life.

HUNTINGTON'S DIS-EASE

This dis-ease results in involuntary muscle movement and mental deterioration. Those who acquire this dis-ease are individuals who have suffered some unpleasant emotional experience in their life. This experience caused them to turn inward on themselves and away from life. They are *shutting themselves off* from their surroundings. The exposed feeling resulted from an unpleasant experience made them want to hide. They now fear to allow themselves out again, to be exposed, in fear that they will get the same *negative response* that they have gotten in the past. Living in this state over a period of time begins to imprint this state within the cells of the body, and thus the body begins to exist in this state: the part of the brain that is associated with producing action starts to close off.

Although this center is prevented from responding, the brain is still receiving. The stimulus is still coming in, yet the person is not willingly allowing a response to go out. This imbalance produces an overload, which therefore causes energy to be forced out, resulting in *involuntary responses*. The soul is stating that if we are not going to respond in life voluntarily, then the response will be taken out of *our will* and become *involuntary*.

Remember that there is not a wrong action or way of responding, as long as the intention is good. Acting is a way of expressing *who we are*, which can never be wrong. The more a person with Huntington's dis-ease can reduce their fear of responding, the more control they will have over their involuntary movements. This dis-ease teaches them that it's OK to respond. Their soul brought on this dis-ease because they now can't hide themselves from responding: it just happens. The control is taken out of their hands. This experience helps them learn to be OK with freely expressing themselves.

The soul learning is that these individuals need to realize that everybody goes through or is exposed to negative emotions. It's part of life, and the only true way to overcome these negative emotions is to face them and find new positive ways to cope through them, until you overcome them. The most important lesson is to not let the fear of the bad stop you from experiencing the good in life. These individuals need to realize that they do have a place in life and should be making that place for themselves.

HYPERTHYRODISM

The cause for this dis-ease in terms of learning is an excessive amount of self-expression. This person is expressing them self too much, to the point that their self or identity is spread too thin and burned out. This type of person feels too compelled to take charge of life. They cannot sit back and let things happen. This action sounds motivating and productive, yet when taken to this degree, one can end up pushing options right out of one's life, because there's no room left for them. Often, by jumping the gun, such people miss many of life's opportunities.

Individuals with hyperthyroidism are tying too hard to identify themselves in the world because of their *insecurity* with their place in it. They try to make a strong place for themselves, so as to stand out. They strive for this, because it makes them feel like somebody. They need to make themselves known in order to feel good.

Their soul learning is to stop proving themselves in life. They spend too much time trying to prove themselves that they burn themselves out. They expect more than they can give. What they do not realize is that what they are easily capable of giving is often more than enough.

HYPOGLYCEMIA

Individuals with hypoglycemia are constantly trying to stabilize themselves. When they cannot get their inner needs meet through external things, they question their self-worth. In response, they spend an enormous amount of time trying to force circumstances in their life to prove otherwise. These individuals are facing an inner crisis of *"Can it be done?"* or *"Can I do well enough?"*

These individuals need to look at themselves in a different light. Their soul learning is to look at who they are within and stop trying to prove themselves externally. True self-worth can only be obtained through an inner perception of oneself. Nothing external will ever be good enough to prove to them what they need to see in themselves.

HYPOTHYROIDISM

Hypothyroidism arises when someone has slowed down their personal self-expression, because of a loss of *self-identity*. These individuals are in conflict between who they are and who they should be. They aren't sure, so they don't express their thoughts, feelings and beliefs. They do not allow themselves to freely express who they are. They keep things bottled up within, which gives them a puffy look. This puffiness symbolizes all of the energy (thoughts, feelings and beliefs) stored in their body that they are not expressing.

These individual's soul learning is to learn to *identify* with themselves, which can only be done through expressing themselves in order to find out who they are. The problem is that they fear this personal expression. The fear is similar to a agoraphobia, where one fears to leave one's house. In this case, they fear to step outside of themselves, yet this is exactly what they need to do.

HYSTERIA

Hysteria occurs when individuals cannot deal with the circumstances they are currently facing. They *over-react* to the situation and as a result create conversion reactions. They use these reactions as a cover they can hide behind, so they do not have to deal with the situation. Because they are having a hard time with what is right in front of them, they use this method as a way to cope with the circumstances that they cannot face. They take measures to the extreme, trying so desperately to overlook the situation that they are in.

Don't think for a minute that they don't realize what they need to face: They do; it is just that they are having a hard time right now. Other individuals should not force them to see what they cannot yet face. This will only cause them to become more hysterical. Their soul learning is to try and learn different coping methods to face these circumstances in their life without over-reacting. And remember that God never gives us more than we can handle, even though it may not seem like it at times.

I

IMPOTENCE

These individuals don't think highly of themselves. That's not because they are impotent, but rather it's the other way around: they have the problem of impotence because they don't think highly enough about themselves in general.

They don't think that they are successful, and they are willing to accept this view of themselves because they aren't sure how to go about being successful. They don't realize that they just have to try and not give up along the way when things get hard, so to speak. These are their challenges in life. They are part of their growing and learning processes. This is the only way they can become successful at anything.

At times they even try to convince themselves that they are happy where they are at, yet this is only because they question whether they can become more of what they want. This uncertainty translates into their sexual life as questioning whether they can *do it*, leading to the problem of impotence. These individuals' soul learning is to think more highly of themselves and have respect for what they can do and who they are. Once this is learned, this dis-ease will exit the body.

INFECTION (BACTERIAL)
(SEE ALSO INFECTION - VIRAL)

Bacterial infections are usually localized within a particular area in the body, where as a viral infection affects the whole body. Bacterial infections are ignited by an external factor, but the match itself is formed inside the person based on their true feelings. When one has allowed an infection to affect their body, it has as well allowed these feelings that they could not tame to take control over them. These negative feelings that are now burning them up is because these negative thoughts and feelings have been stored for too long.

Someone who gets an infection have thoughts and feelings inside that are boiling over. They are trying to control or deal with them and they are not able to. An infection is not an instantaneous thing, though it may appear that way. Rather these negative feelings, which are its ruler, build over time until it gets to a point of overload in which the body must release this build-up. Therefore, an infection arises to create an outlet for the negative thoughts and feelings.

By the time one acquires an infection at the physical level, these inner feelings have festered into a huge boiling point that has more pizzazz than the infection did when the infection started. The individual has held these negative thoughts and feelings inside for too long without letting them out to be exposed. The individual has tried to conceal their thoughts and feelings over a particular circumstance that they just cannot let go of. This concealment has caused these negative feelings to now become an infection.

Having an infection is the way that the body gets a chance to *let off some steam*, so to speak. This is the body's natural defense mechanism to burn off some of the unwanted negative effects of these negative emotions that are out of control, so that they do not do such severe damage to the body.

When one has an infection, the soul learning is to take a look at what has emotionally been ignited for them to understand and *come to terms* with. This is done through facing and then expressing these negative thoughts and feelings to be able to release them and move on.

These individuals also have a mind that is very overindulging. They don't want to miss anything in life. Because they are not satisfied with what is, they always look for more. They jump into everything nose first without thinking. This causes them to take on too many things in their life. They end up losing touch with what it is they need to be doing, because they are so busy just doing something. Being caught up in so many things externally leaves them with less time for inner learning because they are so busy externally doing. This causes them to lose ground with their original intention and purpose in life. From the outside, it looks as if they are in overdrive mode, overexerting their bodies too much. Yet, this overdrive mode is propelled from within. They need to look at what the drive is behind this continual external doing. This dis-ease will slow them down so they can take some time to look at life and get back on track. They need to realize that it is not about how much they do or even how capable they are, as long as they just make themselves available.)

INFECTION (VIRAL)
(SEE ALSO INFECTION - BACTERIAL)

Viral infections affect the whole body rather than a particular area (the latter found with bacterial infections). People who get viral infections have emotional needs that are not met, and the reason those needs are not met is because the people fear being able to get them met. They don't want to have to face possible rejection.

In all cases of infection, buried emotions are festering, but the nature of the problem is different with viral and bacterial infections. Whereas bacterial infections reflect negative emotions that are burning us up, viral infections are caused by emotions that are burning us out.

Viral infections are very self-oriented; they are not circumstantial or as easily overcome. It is a personal problem towards the self, not towards something or someone else. Where as, with bacterial infections the feelings are directed at someone or something. With viral infections anger or negative emotions are not the cause, but rather sad emotions. These people are sad and feel lonely, but they are bringing it on themselves by not allowing their needs to be meet. Those with bacterial infections are denying themselves out of spite. Bacterial infections are anger-motivated. In contrast, viral infections are brought on because these individuals don't feel worthy, so they won't allow their needs to get met.

The overall soul learning for this dis-ease is to realize that everyone experiences rejection. Therefore, by not allowing themselves to receive, these individuals are not allowing love to flow within and around them. Instead they need to learn that they need to express their needs rather than denying them out of fear of rejection.

The soul learning is that putting oneself in a position where one might be rejected is worth it because one might instead actually get one's *needs* meet. The alternative is letting these needs reach the stage of infection by never expressing them and not accepting this love in that is so desperately needed. Rather than continuing to live with these sad and lonely emotions inside, that over time causes one to become burned out, are needs to overcome their fear and learn to express their true feelings letting them out.

INFERTILITY

Those who are infertile are still really deep down within questioning their ability and decision to become a parent. They are indecisive because their underlying issue revolves around the idea that they feel and think that they might not be able to be a successful parent. First, the soul learning is that they have to come to realize that there is no such thing as a *perfect parent*, but at the same time there is. We really are all perfect, doing exactly what we are capable of. We are always doing everything to the best of our ability, and that is indeed perfect.

When there is enough soul growth on both parents' parts, then there is time for expansion through procreation. A new soul is created from the parents' two souls.

All that both of the two parents' souls have or have not learned through eons of generations is passed on to the new soul, the child, to now learn and grow more, to then one day pass on to future generations. When the time is right and both parents are ready, they will indeed conceive. It's important not to force the process, just as God does not force a flower to bloom. Conception happens on its own accord, when all is ready.

INFLAMATION (ACUTE)

A sudden onset of inflammation is caused by an individual's unwillingness to participate in life. They have stopped themselves in the midst of action. When a sudden onset of inflammation arises in our life, we need to look to what we are currently involved in that we just put a halt to. This is where the problem lies. We stopped action that was in progress, thus causing a backup of energy that induced this inflammation. We must go back to that issue or subject and finish our business and let things play out. Even if events seem undesirable, understand that there is a divine intention for them that is necessary. By stopping it from playing through, we are now causing ourselves discomfort.

The reason why one would stop the course of action in the midst of it is because they suddenly questioned whether they are capable enough to continue on. They question their ability in the current situation, wondering whether there might be a possibility of failure, so they stop that action from continuing any further. Yet, they need to not stop things from happening in their life just because it could prove them as incapable; otherwise they will never learn to become capable. If they let this fear of not being capable hold them back, they could remain incapable for the rest of their lives.

Their soul learning is that they need to learn to not stop themselves from being themselves because they are in fear of being incapable. Instead, they need to finish what they started and take that last step in order to come to see themselves as capable. Then and only then, will they be able to believe that they are capable.

INFLUENZA
(SEE ALSO INFECTIONS – VIRAL)

The cause for the flu is similar to any viral infections. It is a case where the body is attacking the body with consequences. *"What you have done to me, you will get back,"* the body is stating. In this case, the individual has failed to care for the body, monitoring its needs and supplying it with the care or love that it needed. In return, the body is rebelling. The effect of this *lack of care* is that the body feels helpless and drained everywhere, as if it is hard to even take another breath, because it requires too much energy. This is done so that the individual can again regain the joy of life after having the pleasure removed. After taking the body and being for granted so long, the hope through this dis-ease is that simple respect for them self will come of it. You could say that those who get the flu are those who aren't taking care of themselves. The flu occurs when an individual is not giving the appropriate attention needed to them self. They end up draining the body of its energy and not making sure that they are supplying it for the demand that they are asking of it. Their soul learning is that they must make sure that their supply always meets their demands.

INSOMNIA

The inability to fall asleep, or to remain sleeping restfully, is the result of an individual's inability to *let go* and let things rest; therefore they can't rest. They constantly worry about something or somebody. They are always thinking about something. They have to make sure things are all set in place as they think they should be, so that they can make sure that things will be OK in their minds. These individuals fear that they will be caught off guard. They feel unsafe. They feel they must be prepared for everything. Either they stay up worrying about everything, trying to think things through, or they don't totally sleep soundly, because even in their sleep state they cannot let things rest.

These individuals think that they must take control to make everything all right. They feel they are responsible for things. They need to realize that we only have so much power, so they must do what they can and then let the rest be in God's hands. These individuals' soul learning is to learn to *let go and let God*. They need to understand that things will happen as they are intended to be. There are no accidents; rather, all experiences are there for learning in order for one to grow. They need to worry less and have more faith that God has things under control.

ITCHING

Itching is brought on when one is in a state of discontentment. They are completely unsettled with certain circumstances in their life. This occurs because they are unable at this time to deal with the situation in their life that is now causing them aggravation. Itching is how they are releasing their *aggravation* from within. Whatever is bothering them within is showing through on the outside. Something has literally *gotten under their skin*. Something has them aggravated and they cannot seem to let it go. It is unsettled in their mind so it gets underneath their skin, so to speak. They are in a state of fear because they are uncertain of the situation, so they want to run, and when you run away from it, you end up running away with yourself. After it gets to a high point, it causes an outbreak, releasing in this case through the skin as itching. Itching is one of the body's natural mechanisms to release excessive energy.

Their soul learning is to look to identify what is causing them to be aggravated and then learn to express and deal with it, rather than holding it in and letting this aggravation build. Then it will no longer be under their skin and the itching will cease.

J

JAUNDICE

This is a common occurrence among newborns which indicates that they are not yet willing to participate in life. They are a little apprehensive about life. They are not content with their surroundings; it seems unsettling to them. These children have entered life with a resistance, so they still have parts of themselves closed off. They have not yet fully opened up to life. Basically, they aren't ready to be here. Yet, they are already here and are being forced to face life, so they are a little upset.

What it boils down to is that because these children have not fully opened up to life, the body is suffering. They are not totally *willing* yet, so their body is unable to be totally functioning. The liver is the organ that commonly suffers because they are angry with the situation that they have been forced to deal with.

Through this experience, the child will acquire their soul learning by realizing that their body is filling with toxicity (anger) and they need to turn that around into love if they want life. The best help that parents and loved ones can offer is pouring in "LOVE" from the outside. This helps the child wake up to life and love.

JOINT INFLAMMATION

(Acute, not long-term)

Inflammation arises due to circumstances in one's life that causes them to be on edge. This occurs because they are over-investing themselves in something, often because they are trying to run from something else. They are trying to run and hide from a current issue at hand in their life right now by involving themselves in many new things.

These people are unhappy with their current circumstances. They desperately want to change them, yet they often try too hard to do so in an inappropriate way. They involve themselves in many new experiences external to themselves, when they need to be looking at and dealing with the current issue at hand in front of them. Then they wouldn't be unhappy with how their life currently is. Instead of running and doing something else in an attempt to avoid this learning, they need to do something about the learning that they now face. Their soul learning is that they need to stop running and start facing.

K

KIDNEY PROBLEMS

These individuals are at a loss for who they are and where they are supposed to be going in life. They have let themselves stay in the back ground, not to be heard for too long. They have learned how to let themselves stuff who they are by not allowing themselves to be spoken for.

These individuals are the type that is not able to let certain things bounce off them so easy; metaphorically this shows through in the kidneys having trouble filtering. What people say about them they really take to heart, even the small things. Any criticism really affects them. They have in a lot of ways become *the image* created of them by others. That is why they are lost with who they are and where they are. Because others have categorized them in certain terms of who they are, that's why they're having trouble with who they are and where they are. Instead of themselves displaying who they really are, they have gotten caught up being what others say they are.

The soul learning is they need to learn to be who they truly are by standing up for what they think and feel, not what others are telling them to be and do. They need to learn from what others have to say, and let the rest bounce off of them so that their kidneys can again filter properly.

KNEE PROBLEMS
(GENERAL)

The knee represents the joint that allows you to move and walk through life. People who have knee problems are having trouble taking a big step in their life right now. They are hesitant to take the leap that life is requiring of them. They tend to be stubborn about sticking to a particular way of doing things. They become unwilling to make adjustments. This inflexibility shows through in the body, in this case the knee. Overall, they need to make some big changes in their life, and they are having trouble.

Ultimately, what ends up happening is that they are not able to freely walk through life without pain or discomfort. This is a reminder to them that they are having trouble taking some particular step and making some changes that they need to address in their life. Pain* is present to remind them of the steps their soul is requiring them to take.

People who acquire knee problems are having trouble adjusting to life's new demands. Yet, the reason they are having trouble taking these steps and making these changes is deeper seated than simple unwillingness or stubbornness to change, as it appears. The reason that one is unwilling to take this step and make this change is because they are lacking confidence in their capabilities in being able to do so. They don't know if they can do it.

Once they get past believing that they can do it, next they question if they will be able to do it well enough. This is a hidden fear of theirs. This fear causes them to become too afraid to take this step. Therefore, they become hesitant and unwilling to endeavor. They will tend to procrastinate. Over time, they become more resistant to taking these steps and making these changes. Ultimately, the reason boils down to them not totally being confident in their capabilities. They question their worth in terms of their ability in action, not internally speaking. *They fear their capabilities in action.* Because of this hidden fear the task of freely accepting change is much more difficult for them.

Their soul learning is to be more flexible in life. They need to accept these changes and take these steps in order for the knee to be relieved of the pain and it can begin to heal and restore health. It is helpful for the individual to look at these changes as a new adventure full of new beginnings. These individuals need to not let their fear of being capable hold them back from being able to experience new things in life. Realize that it is ultimately only by taking the steps and going through these changes that we indeed learn to become capable.

*Remember, pain is always a sign from our soul trying to tell us that we are having trouble learning something. If we did not have pain, we would never stop and pay attention to what our body and soul is trying to tell us.

L

LIVER

Any problems relating to the liver reflect the way an individual feels about them self. These people are really down on themselves. They are unhappy with the environment, the conditions in their life and where their position is in life. Their place to them in life is unknown and their identity is not what they wish it to be.

The liver in dis-ease deals with the individual being angry with themselves for who they are and where they currently stand in life. They deny themselves what they deserve out of life. This is their punishment to themselves for not being what they feel they should be. They commonly compare themselves with others for this judgment.

These people feel that they do not have what it takes to *do* and *be* in life, so therefore they are angry with themselves about it. Eventually, they begin to destroy themselves over it. The liver is unable to filter the overload of toxic emotions, which has become negative energy. These toxic emotions reflect the anger that they have for themselves.

These people need to learn to love themselves for who they are, not *what* they are. The focus needs to become internal. They avoid this internal reference, because they cannot escape from these emotions there. But the answers are there. They need to see who they are, not defined by the world outside of themselves, but defined by *themselves*. They need to learn to let that true self out, giving themselves a chance to become and do something.

Their soul learning is to love them self for who they are, instead of trying to be somebody they're not. If they continue to try to live up to the standards of others they will continue to be unhappy and angry with themselves, because they are trying to base who they are on the standards of others instead of themselves.

LOU GEHRIG'S DIS-EASE

People with this dis-ease rapidly deteriorate because they have decided to shut themselves off from receiving the things they need out of life. They have closed themselves in to block out the outside world. Those who face this dis-ease have had experiences in their present life that have induced some hurt(s). Now, they do everything they can so that they don't have to experience such hurt again. They have handled the troubles of the past, yet they are sure to not adventure into new experiences that could possibly lead to emotional tragedy or hurt. So, they emotionally close down. They have this technique of shutting themselves down and not letting in life. Yet, this puts them in danger by not being able to receive what they need to sustain them self. They can only equally receive in energy from life equivalently to what they have given out.

By withdrawing themselves from life, they end up closing off the energy of life; therefore their body does not receive the energy it needs. At first it is hard to notice directly on the body itself; rather it is apparent in their lifestyle. They begin to refrain from life, as if they are letting things pass them by. By them not letting life in, they restrict energy; therefore things are unable to transpire for them in their life. After a period of time, life cannot go on without adequate energy coming in, so the body suffers and creates this dis-ease.

They shut themselves off from receiving out of life because they are in fear that they will have to face that particular emotion that was tragic to them again. They shut themselves down in an attempt to avoid any more possible related emotional tragedy. An individual who has acquired this dis-ease, as with all dis-eases, was born with this soul learning in their genetics, in this case long overdue from their ancestors. In this lifetime, their soul has been focused on presenting them opportunities (experiences in life) in which they could have learned to allow themselves to take on life and the new hurts that may accompany it. But if not learned, then the soul learning reaches its peak and *will* now be addressed and learned through the dis-ease. The soul learning for these individuals is for them to get to a point where they can again allow themselves to experience life at all costs, risking new emotional hurts. This is necessary in order for them to be able to live, learn and grow.

LOW IMMUNE SYSTEM

When one has a low immune system, whether starting from birth, or acquired somewhere along their journey through life, the soul learning is *standing up for themselves*. The immune system genetically consists of who we are as a person. All of the strengths, immunities and weaknesses (areas needing further soul growth) that we have or have not acquired, both from our ancestors and the learning (or lack therefore) that we have or haven't obtained in our individual life thus far make up the unique person that we are today. Therefore, when we do not take a stand for who we are, our immune system is sure to weaken, because we are denying ourselves.

When people are born with immune problems it signifies that upon coming into this life their ancestors were not yet able to fight for who they were. They were not able to stand for themselves to a point that now the next generation will come into life set up with the opportunity to deal with this soul learning. If they acquired immune problems later in life, then this would signify that the individual probably came into this life with this learning to stand up for themselves, and was first offered learning through life experiences to learn it before having to go through acquiring this dis-ease.

Individuals with a low immune system are not eager to make a place for themselves in life. They have already let so much of it pass them by, to the point now that it is biologically affecting their immune system. Their soul learning is to come out of their shell within, which is their hiding place. Through the process of this dis-ease it teaches them how to fight for life, thereby learning how to *stand up for them self.*

LUNG PROBLEMS

Individuals who face problems with their lung(s) in general have too many emotions that they always have to try to figure out how they are going to deal with them. They are the type that gets involved with trying to take care of other people and their feelings too often, and what ends up happening is that their own feelings never get taken care of, and then they wonder *"Why is this happening to me?"*

Their soul learning is to learn to confront the situations in their life when their feelings are being stepped on and taken advantage of, rather than avoiding them and just dealing with them within. They are literally smothering themselves. Their problem is that they spend too much time dealing with things, taking on the responsibilities of others and end up keeping their feelings within them. Instead, it is time that they need to let other people deal with their own responsibilities and start taking care of their own needs, expressing their feelings and no longer letting others take advantage of them.

LYMPHATIC PROBLEMS
(GLANDS AND NODES)

Any lymphatic problems are related to the immune system. The immune system is a part of the body that is known as the *adaptation system*. This adaptation system consists of all of the learnings acquired throughout all of our lineage, known as our strengths or immunities. It also includes the learnings that have not been acquired through our lineage; these are known as our weaknesses, areas that still need learning. Problems arise because the *individual* is giving up their fight. They are not standing up for themselves. They are not letting themselves fight for who they are, thus they are fading away.

Specific problems of the lymph glands and nodes indicate *toxic emotions about self.* There is a part of them self that is not happy with who they are at this time, and with their place in life, so they are now going through a stage of giving up. They are losing themselves with life, letting them self drift away by not standing up for who they are as a person.

They are lacking self-confidence and worth. They feel that they don't count; therefore they are not standing up for themselves like they need to be. Rather, they are hiding, staying quiet. These specific stored emotions about themselves that they are not standing up for have turned toxic, thereby resulting in lymph problems. There soul learning is to learn to stand up for themselves and who they are, not letting themselves fade away, but rather shine!

M

MENENGITIS

Through this dis-ease, the infection itself takes over and becomes the expression of one's feelings that have not had a chance to be heard. Infection is present within the body when one is overwhelmed about a particular soul learning that is not being faced or dealt with by them. These people need to get something off of their chest and they need help doing it, so through this infection the body is helping them release some of these negative thoughts and feelings. Through this illness they are able to learn better techniques for letting their feelings out as opposed to letting them build and backfire within.

Individuals with this dis-ease have faced their life with an inner disgust about them self, and this attitude prevails in their life. People with this illness feel lost in life. They don't know where to focus their energy. They truly can't find their place. They often question, *"What am I doing here?"* These individuals' soul learning is to take time and discover their place and purpose in life, instead of looking to blame themselves or others for this blank question. Questioning their ability and sitting in the back seat in life is going to get them nowhere. They need to realize that they are strong enough to make a place for themselves, and that it will work if they put forth the effort. God has a divine place and purpose awaiting each and every one of us.

MENOPAUSAL PROBLEMS

Women who face menopausal problems are having a difficult time with the transition of their womanhood. This transition of being a women involves an inner conflict about the meaning of being a woman. What it once used to mean to them is now changing its meaning as a whole as they enter a new stage in their life. Their role as a woman is now again changing. They are facing problems making this transition. They face inner conflict on how they think they should be, appear, act and so forth as a women at this new stage in their life. Their body in turn faces some internal turmoil over the conflict in changing their perspectives to now learning new aspects of what it means to be a women.

What these women need to do is to sit back, relax and try to let their bodies lead them through. These individuals should not force the body to do something it is not yet able or comfortable doing. These individuals soul learning is to take the time and space they need to make this transition until they are able to adapt into their full potentiality of woman-ness – what being a women means to them. They need to be all of who they are as a woman and let it come naturally and freely. They must let go of what they think they should be according to standards of society and *be the woman they are.*

Surely this time will bring about some conflict in making this transition; adjustments will have to be made. Yet, what is important to realize is to not focus on them too much; rather let them happen freely on their own. Trying to fit into all of these roles and positions of what is involved in being a woman all at once becomes overwhelming to all levels of our being: mentally, emotionally, spiritually and physically. The best way to approach this crucial emotional time is to let things happen naturally in their own time, conforming to the adjustments life requires when necessary. Giving our self and body the time and space it needs to make this transition is the best thing we can do to help ourselves through this time.

MIGRAINE HEADACHES

Migraine headaches are brought about by an extreme overload of mental energy. One has thought about something so much and cannot *see* how this something in their life or their place in life is ever going to work out or happen. They have thought this out in their mind and cannot see it working, to the point that the brain goes into overload, to such a degree that biologically they end up not even being able to take in any more stimuli, such as light or noise, without inducing more pain. This is because the energy has been so built up and blocked up due to the individual not having understanding that they cannot take in anything else, without first getting some placement about the situation at hand.

Sleep is often helpful because the subconscious gets a chance to help bring understanding to the conscious mind through subliminal messages, that when we wake up we refer to as our dreams. The soul learning for these individuals is that they need to realize that they do not need to be so closed-minded. They need to be less analytical and become more creative and spontaneous.

Instead of being on a merry-go-round with this repetitious thinking, which is the reason why the migraine headache came to begin with, they need to learn to be more open to other possibilities to help them to get out of this vicious cycle. By opening up to these new ideas and possibilities, they will be able to come to a conclusion so that they are able to put things to rest.

MONONUCLEOSIS

An individual who has mononucleosis is not expressing themselves at this time in their life. Their emotions are closed down and reserved. They have many stored emotions and feelings locked deep inside that are not on the burner for discussion. Someone or something has really upset them, and they are storing their feelings within about it.

People who have mono are people who have a part of themselves locked away. They have tried to keep a specific part of themselves that they don't like about themselves hidden, yet it has reached a boiling point resulting in this dis-ease, and they can no longer deny it. Acquiring mononucleosis is the way that the body can release all of the frustration that has been kept locked in. Much pain is unleashed at all levels, mentally, emotionally, spiritually and physically, with the onset of this dis-ease.

One who has mono has a body that is burning up inside because of this rejection of self, by self. This is why it is common to have the Effect be on the liver. The fury involved will dictate the degree of damage to the liver during this virus. They are not able to accept a part of them self, so they deny this part. This soul needs to learn to be free and open with all of themselves, all of who they are, not hiding any parts of themselves. Their soul learning is to learn to accept all of themselves for who they really are, and stop denying their self. They need to learn to express their thoughts and feelings in all cases at all times, instead of holding back and living in frustration from not expressing who they really are and how they really feel.

MOUTH SORES – CANKER SORES

Anyone who develops any mouth sores inside or out is someone who is holding back from expressing or saying something that they need to be. The reason that they are not expressing is because they're afraid to, afraid of the results being unfavorable.

Their soul learning is that they need to realize that things are not always going to be favorable in life. And by holding themselves back from what might be an unfavorable outcome or result, ultimately, they are holding their souls back from what they are supposed to be doing. Not only is it hurting them by not saying or expressing it, it is also hurting the other person(s) to whom they need to express it, because the other person(s) need to hear it as well, for their soul learning. They were not there by accident either. If the sores are inside, it's a deeper issue of discussion, while if they are on the outside it's a surface issue of discussion.

MULTIPLE SCLEROSIS

People with Multiple Sclerosis are individuals with a lot of feelings. Because they are feeling-oriented, this puts a lot of stress on their nervous system. They are always *going above and beyond the call of duty*. They outdo themselves. They put themselves on overload and end up running their bodies down, because they are overdoing their true capacity. They are always trying to be more and do more than they are truly capable of. They feel inadequate at their core, and that is why they *over do*, in order to make up for that feeling. They create undue stress in their lives by forcing things to happen, because it's a way to *make them feel better*. They need to realize that there is no need to outdo them self to shine – they already do!

They are always trying to force things to work the way they think they should be. Yet, because they are too busy trying to enforce their own plans, they end up closing themselves off from other opportunities. They must understand that things are as they are for a reason; they are divine. They need to sit back and realize that they cannot do everything. They must remember, *no man is an island alone*. They need to learn a little more of *"let go and let God."*

Overdoing anything, even out of positive intention, can lead to destruction. The soul learning is to not overdo, and through the process of MS this soul learning will come to be learned. Through this dis-ease process one *will* learn to not overdo, because this dis-ease enables them from doing.

By learning to not always overdo and learning to take life easier, then eventually these onsets of multiple sclerosis will subside because they have learned not to overdo or force things in their life. At this point they will come to realize that who they are is good enough – even great. They don't need to try to be more than they are.

MUSCULAR DYSTROPHY

This dis-ease teaches the individual a respect for life. Life is giving them a calling because they are not willing to grow on their own. They don't mind just *existing*, but they fear *living*. Yet, if they are not going to get with the program, the program is going to get to them. Thus, if they don't go after life, life will consume them.

These individuals have not lived life outside of themselves: rather, they just existed in themselves. They stopped participating in life, so they begin to lose themselves, who they are. As much as you need to go within in order to get in touch with who you are, to know who you are, it is equally important to go without to look externally to see and reflect who you are. We must do both to see and understand the whole of self. So, because *they aren't applying themselves* they don't know themselves. If we don't apply our self in life then we are not able to feel and become worthy of life.

The soul learning is that by not participating in life and only existing within themselves, over time they lose their self, who they are. Because they are in fear of feeling not worthy, they don't apply themselves. This fear causes them to end up not really knowing themselves. By not applying them self in life, the living in life will become limited, until they can wake up and see that not applying themselves is causing more trouble than facing their fear of being inadequate or unworthy. In fact, it is only by doing in life that we learn to be adequate and then we can feel worthy about ourselves internally and externally.

N

NAUSEA

When one develops nausea it is because they are way overdoing them self. They have bitten off more than they can truly handle. They may be the type that occasionally does this or commonly does this. If nausea is something that occurs often for them it is because they are constantly questioning if they really like who they are. To make themselves feel better about themselves they over invest them self in many things, thereby putting too many demands on them self. This is done because the individual questions whether they are important. They wonder if they can flourish, so this is why they try to outdo to prove themselves.

Their soul learning is that they need to learn to like themselves for who they are. They don't need to do any more, putting excessive demands on themselves, to be important and flourish. They need to realize that they are as important as each individual on this earth is, with a uniquely important purpose that their soul has the details set for them to divinely accomplish.

NECK

Individuals who have neck problems is related to one who is bottling up their energy. The *old stiff neck*. They hesitate to freely allow their self to *express* what they really think and feel. They are holding back. This causes the neck to carry around bottled-up energy that is eventually going to be indicative of problems. To have balanced energy we need to express the way we feel and think no matter the results. There must be an equal amount of energy going in as coming out, at all times, at all levels, for overall balance and health.

By storing their energy they are not allowing themselves to really express who they are. They are actually forcing their energy or power level to stay in and not demand its attention. This creates a weak power level or personality. This is indicative of one who is on guard and not allowing things to freely happen.

When we block energy in our body, we are also blocking energy from freely coming in our life; thus we are stopping things from happening around us. Also, by not expressing who we really are, we are not putting the attention on what we really think or feel, our opinion, which is indicative of a weak personality. Thus, it is not just a matter of not opening a doorway, but rather we are actually closing doorways in our life by bottling up our energy and staying so self-oriented instead of sharing our opinions and truths with others.

The soul learning for these individuals is to appropriately demand their feelings and thoughts to be expressed, no matter what others think or how they feel. They need to work on allowing them self to freely express themselves. Not only will they feel better, their life will change. By not expressing their true thoughts and feelings, the energy stays blocked, in this case in their neck, not freely flowing – expressing who they are.

NERVE PROBLEMS

The nervous system is the part within the body that carries and sends all messages to and from the brain. It is the highway for transmission. When somebody has a problem with the nerves it is because the highway has been distorted, due to such things as stress, accidents or dis-ease.

In the case of stress, the brain is sending excessive messages via the nervous system, which causes it to become overloaded, carrying too many messages at one time. This is not just a matter of excessive messages, but excessive *mixed messages*. This is due to the individual excessively thinking, which is triggered by the various stresses in their lives.

When we are stressed-out or edgy, our nerves are energized. At this point we are not content and cannot seem to pacify ourselves. We are unable to calm down or relax. We often get like this because of certain circumstances that we are unable to understand, at the time, the reason for it. This uncertainty instills a sense of fear that is overwhelming. In this state the individual is worried because they don't know what life has yet to hold for them. They fear the next step.

When there are nerve problems with the actual nerves or function of the nerves themselves, there is a bigger issue working behind the scenes. These individuals have a set way of living that has gotten them into this, not just certain conditions or circumstances that arose, but rather many.

They have a mindset that is questioning their self worth, causing nerve problems. They battle with an inner turmoil that they fight and face every day. They face anxiety about internal conditions, as well as the stresses due to external conditions. They are always sending their own personal messages to themselves to keep going and doing. Everyday they have themselves on overdrive inside, which is as well often seen on the outside. They need to calm down and learn that there is a divine plan and no matter how much worrying they do, this divine plan knows exactly what's needed for their soul learning.

Nerves are excited by emotions. These emotions are questions that we have about our self and life. People with any nerve problems are questioning themselves in some area of their life.

The soul learning is that there are things that we do have control over, but as well there are many things we do not have control over, so this lack of control brings with it an feeling of uncertainty both internally and externally, not knowing what's coming next. This is where we need to keep in mind that the one thing we do have control over is ourselves, how we will and will not act and react. We are only so capable, and there are many times that although we think we are capable to handle things, we are not. Know that God has a divine plan for each and every one of us, and God doesn't give us anymore than we can handle. It is time to let go of the things in our life that we are having trouble with and let God take care of the rest. Trusting, believing and knowing!

NEURALGIA

These individuals don't know how to say the word *no*. They get themselves involved in more than they can handle in life. They are not hesitant enough. They jump into things too easily. They end up becoming too self-accepting of the demands of life and others that can never be met.

This either stems back to childhood from a parent, or currently from somebody close to them who expects and demands a lot from them, actually more than the individual is truly capable to handle themselves, but they would never say no. They spend their life always trying to meet demands that are impossible. Today their interpretation of their life is, *If I am able, I am good enough.*

If we are always seeking the approval of others, or trying to meet the demands of others, in order to feel good enough about ourselves, then we will not ever feel good enough about ourselves. Our own standard is the *only* measurement that we should be using to display the unique individuals that we are.

Their soul learning is to come to see that we are good enough just as we are.

How good we are is not based on what we can or cannot do. This is not an external measurement, but rather an internal one. We are all unique individuals here to share with each other our various perspectives of life, from different viewpoints, to whole different perspectives.

NEURITIS

This dis-ease is related to one's learning of self-worth. These individuals live in constant inner turmoil over whether or not they are good enough. They are always running themselves down by trying to *over-do* their self to prove to others how much they can do. They have an inner fight to prove to themselves that they are good enough; this is what they are always striving for. They are trying to prove to everybody but them self, and this is the cause of their inner turmoil. This dis-ease comes about because the nerves are on overload inside. They may look relaxed on the outside, but they are really not relaxed on the inside. Through the process of having this dis-ease they will be forced.

These people question themselves. They always doubt their ability in life and live on edge, therefore always activating their nerves. Nerves run on emotions, and the more they get upset the more the nerves will become inflamed. All of these emotions are questions they have about themselves. These individuals' soul learning is to stop questioning themselves and their abilities. They need to focus on their availability, not their capability.

O

OBESITY

Obesity arises when an individual is not allowing a proper flow of energy in and out of the body. All things in life abide by the basic law of physics that there must be an equal amount of energy going in as well as coming out, in order to have a balance. So, to have a body in balanced proportion, our energy must be balanced at all the levels. We take energy in, through everything that we see, hear, smell, touch and experience, not just through what we taste or eat. As with food and drink, the process of elimination is easy to see. But, from the other senses, "Where does the energy go?" Think about it. Where do you think all the energy that we take in from these other ways goes if there is no elimination? In all that we have seen, heard, smelled and experienced, we took in energy, but if we did not equally express out what we took in through our thoughts, feelings, beliefs and actions, it stays stuck within.

Individuals with obesity are having trouble with a proper flow of energy going out within their lives. This stems from old emotional hurts. These old hurts have caused the individual to feel insecure with expressing himself or herself. Because of this insecurity, they withdraw from being active participants in life. Past actions have led them to believe that life is unsafe for them to *freely express who they are, that is, what they think, feel and believe*, and now they choose to not fully participate in life in fear of a negative emotional feedback related to these old hurts.

Whether the emotion is ridicule, shame or lack of worthiness, etc. , most of all they fear *failure*. They hold back so they don't have to fail. This is truly key. *They decided to not engage in life.* They have let things pass them by because of fear based on past experiences. They stay in too much of a safety zone.

People who are obese are desperately crying from within because their emotions are not met and not heard, and in their mind they can't be fixed. So, one way that they try to supplement their emotional hurts is commonly with food. This method is only a temporary fix for creating a worse situation that goes from a little weight gain to obesity. People who are obese should not focus on food, because the food is not the true cause why they are obese. The reason that these people are eating too much is because they are trying to satisfy emotions that are trapped inside.

The soul learning for obesity is to learn how to deal with these emotions (old hurts) that are holding one back from engaging in life, learning to let go and move on. One needs to put them self back out there in life, freely expressing who they are. They need to confront situations that they face instead of avoiding their feelings and stuffing them. They need to express their feelings, speaking up for what they feel and who they are, even though it may be uncomfortable. Their body is telling them that it is a necessity. Otherwise, they will stay stuck, stagnant, passing by opportunities that life gives them because they fear to act and face these emotions. What they need to do is to **take action** regardless – go beyond the past hurts. This is the only true way to get past them. Not acting restricts our flow of energy, which leads to obesity.

If we want to keep the body in balanced proportion, we must properly manage our energy, not only by paying attention to the physical level, such as food management and physical exercise, but also and equally important is managing our energies mentally, emotionally, and spiritually, by freely expressing our thoughts, feelings and beliefs.

OSTEOPOROSIS

Osteoporosis is related to one denying themselves their needs from life. They are no longer putting themselves out there in life to get their needs met. They are no longer choosing to play in the game of life. People with this dis-ease often have a conditioned mindset that they are *getting older*. They carry the idea that they are unable to do what they used to do. This mindset is conditioned by society in many ways. Having this mindset particularly causes one to lose their personal drive within.

At this point in their life where the dis-ease has set in, instead of staying young and free within their hearts, they have started to give up and have begun to let life take them over. They begin to dwindle away by no longer fighting for their position in life. They see themselves as if *their time has passed*. They truly need to regain themselves to help themselves with this dis-ease, or to stop the progression of it.

At this point they have let the dis-ease take them over because they have questioned their place in life too much, for too long. When they no longer see a place for themselves in life, this leads them to begin to question whether or not they **count**. They truly want to have a place, but yet they don't think that there is one for them anymore, and they surely do not try to fight for this placement, rather, they just sit back and often let it go by. They need to find a purpose again and let themselves dive into life, rather than sitting back on the sidelines and being swallowed up by it. This is why it is important for them to find themselves a new goal or purpose for themselves in life.

All individuals can fight for their purpose in life. We should never slow down and let life take us over, until eventually we are no longer here. By letting this happen to our self, we end up spending the last years of our life not living life as we once were enjoying, but rather existing. This soul learning is to *never stop living before our time.* We do count to this world and the world does indeed have a place for us, if we will only accept it and take the step to discover it.

P

PANIC DISORDER

With this dis-ease one needs to go back to the past to help them with the present, so they then can get on with their future. These individuals in the past have been through many overwhelming traumatic emotional experiences. The degree or how many traumatic experiences one has been through will determine how often, and how many *panic attacks* one would have, as well as the degree of the panic attack itself. This has left them now in this state of fear, a fear that feels like at any time they could get caught off guard about some unpleasant experience or about something or somebody at any time. These extreme negative experiences from the past are constantly being triggered in their daily lives. These experiences are still going on because during the time of the trauma they went into a state of shock within, which left them emotionally frozen in that time and place, where the emotional traumas took place. They were not able to go through it because they did not know how to deal with it or express it at the time.

The feeling comes upon them suddenly; that's why it's called a panic attack. For most, they are unaware of why they come on. Yet the answer is there: something just occurred that triggered thoughts and feelings associated with the negative emotions they experienced during the trauma. Every time they experience any thoughts and feelings that are similar to the thoughts and feelings they felt during the trauma, they will most likely go into a panic attack. These can be few or many.

These individuals need to get past these fears so that they can fully go on with their life. Just telling them to get over it and move on to the future is not going to work. Yes, this is indeed what we want to accomplish, but in order to get to the future, they have to go back to the past and face the trauma and let themselves go through those feelings. At the time of the trauma, they went into shock within, like freezing. This is a defense mechanism to not have to deal because they could not handle it at the time. So ultimately they never really finished going through the experience. Now they need to face the traumatic experience and those feelings that they have been trying to avoid dealing with, and deal with them. This is the only way to end the panic attacks.

Every time they go through a panic attack they do everything they can to get rid of that feeling, often resorting to extreme measures of taking drugs and even suicide. Yet, what they need to do is stop running from it. It will never go away. In fact, not dealing with these emotions is what has brought them to this extreme of panic, and it will only get worse. They need to *face the feeling* head on. And when that feeling comes on that tells them that things are not ok they must learn to tell them selves that everything *is* OK, that there is a divine plan.

Their soul learning is that they need to continue to go through life's experiences headed their way and not back out, but rather face them. They need to use what they have learned from these experiences and turn these learnings into their strengths. When they encounter new experiences that bring about these thoughts, feelings and fears, they need to face them, and then move on. They are missing too much of life. To face the feelings and fears of the past, they need to start letting go of those negative emotions that have turned into fear and replace them with new feelings and emotions for the future.

First, they need to start by observing their thoughts, feelings and beliefs as they arise, asking them self, "What thoughts and feelings were going through their mind just prior to the rise of the panic attack?" They need to identify with these thoughts, feelings and fears now, in order to face them. Ultimately, by facing these fears in the present, it will help them overcome these fears from the past and catch the new feelings and fears from happening.

When this panic attack presents itself, being triggered in this case by an experience of rejection. By letting this fear hold us back and staying frozen in this state, then things in our life will not be able to move freely. Therefore, we will miss many opportunities in life. We are ultimately holding our own selves back because of our own fears. If we walk through those fears, despite the reminders they bring to us of the traumatic past experiences that we have been through, then we will be able to overcome our fears, prevent the panic attacks from occurring and therefore starting to allow things to happen for us.

PARALYSIS

Paralysis is usually of sudden onset due to a particular incident. Those who acquire paralysis are those individuals that are rejecting their life as it currently is. They are internally not wanting and accepting the opportunity that they have been faced with in their life right now. They do not want to deal with the cards that life has laid out for them, so they try to ignore it.

Paralysis is sort of a payback as a result of one's resistance to face life. They will be frozen or stuck in that time and space that they did not want to deal with; this way they will have to face it. It is truly better if they learn to accept what life has brought their way, and each day to welcome their circumstances of life. Realize that all life experiences are necessary for their soul's growth.

The soul learning is to participate in the game of life rather than choosing to close ourselves down and ignore what life has laid before us. Ultimately, we can never really ignore it. It will catch up with us eventually, so it is better to learn it now than later, because later unfortunately means worse, in this case, leading to paralysis in order to acquire this learning.

PARASITES

There are different types of parasites, slightly different in character, yet all dealing with the same issue. Parasites literally eat one away. They eat or take all the nutrients in ones body that it needs in order to grow. They take away our life force. Those who have parasites are commonly children with little *will* to live. They have little fighting strength for their life. What this dis-ease requires of them is to fight for their life, to fight the parasites for their position in life. They have little will and stamina, which makes this battle difficult. In fact, this is how they acquired the parasites in the first place. They had little will to live so it left room for others (parasites) to come in and take their position in life. They tend to do this in other areas of their life as well, where they let others take them over. Instead of standing up for their truths, their feelings, thoughts and beliefs - and taking control of their own lives, they have allowed others to take control.

Children who commonly acquire this dis-ease do not think very highly of themselves; thus they think little is possible in life for them. They have a low self-esteem, having little ambition to want to live or strive for life. They seem to have no big short-term goals, let alone long-term goals, to focus their energy on. This gives them no strong *will* to live. They need to learn to stand up and fight for themselves in life. The hope or intention of this dis-ease is to teach them to fight for a position or *right for life.*

Their soul learning is to first learn that they have the *right* to life as much as anybody else. Then they need to focus on learning to take a stand for their position or place in life. This will help them build their self-esteem and open them up to the possibilities that are available for them, thus giving them something to strive for.

PARKINSON'S DISEASE

People develop this dis-ease because they no longer think that they fit or *count* in life. As a result, they just put the brakes on inside, so to speak. When they start to close down emotionally and mentally, eventually biologically they actually close down their secretion of dopamine; a hormone that releases positive feelings and thoughts. They are letting life pass them by, rather than jumping into life. They hide behind life because it is too much to jump into. Deep within they want to jump into life, yet they fear whether there is a *place* for them and whether they are still good enough. They question whether they can live up to the standards of life, ultimately according to their own standards of life.

These people have traveled through life with this inner feeling of not *counting*, of questioning whether they are able to live up to life standards and where do they fit in life. At a younger age it is easier to deal with this, yet over time as one gets older, all these hidden feelings aren't as easy to cover up. They can no longer cover up their inner feeling of inadequacy by performing in life. Now the issue begins to surface more and they cannot control it or stop it.

These individuals' soul learning is that they need to realize and accept that they do *count*, no matter what they are or are not doing. This dis-ease inhibits them from doing to give them time to see themselves without a performance act, rather just their *true self*. They also need to realize that they can jump into life: even in their condition there is a place for them. There is a place for everybody in life.

PNEUMONIA

Those who develop pneumonia are dealing with a lot of congested emotional energy. The point at which pneumonia sets in is when the individual's condition has reached an overload of emotional distress that has not been brought forth for them to deal with and/or express it.

Those that acquire pneumonia frequently carry a nature about them in which they are caught in a vicious emotional cycle. They have been faced with an emotional crisis that affected them and they won't bring themselves to express it. Emotional energy not being expressed becomes trapped and can eventually, in this case of this soul learning, causing pneumonia.

These individuals don't express their emotional distress because it is not in their nature to. They don't feel they should burden anybody, or that they deserve to put their problems on somebody else. They don't see themselves as having a right, so they keep it in.

Within this soul learning they need to realize that everybody has a *right* to express what they feel, think and believe – who they are. We are all equal. This includes both are strengths and weaknesses. This is what makes up the whole person. We could not understand things in life if we did not experience both the positive and negative aspects of them. *Who we are* is made of our thoughts, feelings and beliefs, and by not expressing them we are denying the essence of our soul. This denial leads to illness, in this case pneumonia.

POLIOMYELITIS

This dis-ease is caused because of a resistance on the individual's part to accept life and the true intentions for their life. They are not calling out to life, wanting to be a part of it. They don't fear life and they need to. They need to worry about their life. **Value** is the key in this learning process. Learning to value not just life, but their life.

This dis-ease can be fought if there is a willing participant to fight the battle. It's a test of strength. This dis-ease is the ultimate wake-up call for life. They have an unwillingness to let themselves prosper in life. They deny themselves from getting the requirements needed for growing and living. Denying their self is a way that they punish themselves, because they are not satisfied with *who* they are. Ultimately, they are disappointed in themselves.

The soul learning for these individuals is that they need to see the light. Their learning is to start by building their self confidence and *self-worth*. How they are able to do this is by discovering who they are and what they really want out of life. Then convincing them self to start trying to obtain that **today** and each and every day. This will help lead them to find a place for themselves in life that will bring to them much happiness within themselves.

PREMENSTRUAL SYNDROME

Premenstrual symptoms occurs as estrogen levels begin to decrease prior to one's monthly cycle. This hormone is a representation of their feminine self. As this hormone level changes a woman suddenly questions her feminine self. She does not know how to deal with these surges of misplaced emotions. If there are any questions that she carries within related to her femininity, she will be more likely to question herself during this time. Many female problems to begin with are prevalent because of insecurities about their womanhood. These questions of one's femininity during this time stir the nervous system, thus emotions begin to rise and become aggravated. As a result, premenstrual reactions occur. Women who have premenstrual syndrome are having trouble trying to change and adjust to this new adaptation. They need to realize that as life changes, so do we, and this includes our feminine role.

Often during these times women are extra-sensitive to anything that may seem critical of their feminine self. These uncontrollable emotions and mood swings are very common among women who are questioning their femininity. They question whether they are doing good enough as a woman. Women may try to spend time trying to outdo themselves either in certain areas in their life, or in general. Therefore, women who commonly suffer with premenstrual syndrome are women who spend their lives overdoing things in attempts to prove their worth, in order to answer the question that they are in question of, *"Are they good enough as a women?"* These individuals need to spend time in search of *proving to themselves* their own worth as a woman, and nobody can do this for them but them.

Their soul learning is to stop questioning whether they are good enough as a women and rather honor who they are as a woman, looking at what they have accomplished, not only for themselves, but what they have been able to do for others by being the woman that they are.

PROSTATE PROBLEMS

Prostate problems usually occur later in a man's life. This happens about the time he begins to feel unhappy with himself. He doesn't think or feel he can do what he use to do. So he in turn stops doing things he used to do. Overall he thinks and feels that this marks his manhood, holding him back from doing things that he used to do, *what it means to be a man*, in his terms. He doesn't see him self as successful in life, nor does he think that he appears successful. Here is where the real problem comes in. He likes things to *look perfect*: any imperfections he tries to cover up. And now as he is getting older his manhood is not what it used to be in his eyes, so whenever any imperfection shows through an outbreak will arise or increase. If the individual has a big issue with his male role, this can lead to cancer.

This dis-ease is another dis-ease of conscious evolution that is on the rise now because the *male role* has changed and is still changing in our world today. What it once meant to be *a man* has changed. The male position in the home is no longer just the provider, but as well the nurturer. For example, men are learning that it is ok to cry. In other words, since we have been children and were told that boys should not cry, that's like telling them to not use a part of their brain function to express their feelings. We have been conditioned to believe that our emotions make us weak, when it is really quite the contrary; they give us strength. This is because we are actually using more of our brain, because *our emotions come from our brain*. These are emotions that men didn't deal with before, yet now life is demanding it of them And they are having a hard time balancing their emotions.

His soul learning is to come to this balance and *become happy with him self for who he is and what he has accomplished*, and then the prostate problem will over time abate. Remember this dis-ease did not happen over night, so don't expect it to be gone over night. This is true with any long-standing dis-eases. He needs to learn that life's demands are tough and he is doing a good job dealing with it. He needs to stop spending so much time being disappointed within him self for not succeeding at being a perfect model – be mindful that we are all learning.

PSORIASIS
Individuals with psoriasis are those who have a irritation going on within themselves. These individuals live with a constant irritation about their self-worth. They are irritated over their performance in life. They are particularly not pleased with the expectations that they have set for themselves, and have failed to make. Yet, the one thing that they should keep in mind when they push further to succeed is that maybe they need to alter their unrealistic goals and standards that they have set for themselves. Because they set really high goals for what they expect of themselves in comparison to what they actually may be able to do, they are always in constant struggle to meet these demands. If they are unable to meet these demands, then they

view themselves as not adequate or good enough. At these particular times, when things prove to point at feelings of inadequacy, they will notice a flare-up in their psoriasis.

These individuals' soul learning is to not judge adequacy on their self-performance. They need to look at their self from within, rather than from without. By learning to connect with who they are, rather than focusing on how they should appear, this will teach them to slow down and not feel so compelled to prove themself.

R

RASH

A rash arises from a bothered emotional state of being. The individual is bothered by someone or something in their life that has gotten under their skin, so to speak. Because they are not able to forget about it, it stays within to build and fester. They have a one-track mind about the situation that they hold in and let build. This is a way for them to close themselves off from the person or thing that is bothering them. Yet, it is not able to stay closed in forever; it has to have a way out, a release, and so it does in the form of a rash.

A rash can immediately develop from the onset of an unpleasant experience. A continual repeat of a rash is in relation to something or someone that is not new, but rather an ongoing situation.

For example, let's say about eight years ago an individual experienced their dog being attacked by another dog in their backyard next to the lilac trees. So, now when they are around, or come in contact with, lilac trees, they have a reaction to them. Although it seems like it is the lilac tree that caused this reaction, the lilac tree is only the trigger. The cause for the outbreak is really the memory of their dog being hurt eight years ago near the lilac trees.

Food-related intolerances that create a rash are related to the food being linked to the specific emotion that they experienced which was unpleasant at the time they were eating or around that particular food. Therefore, every time they eat or are around that specific food it triggers that unpleasant emotion from the past, thus inducing a reaction, which in this case is a rash.

These individuals soul learning is to be more open-minded in generalthey need to see the unpleasant experience as necessary, divine and for a particular reason. Then the experience will no longer bother or irritate them, the rash can then alleviate.

RHEUMATOID ARTHRITIS

The inflammation, character of rheumatoid arthritis is caused by one's resistance to the flow of energy in their life. They are unhappy with the current circumstances in which they are involved, so they are trying to stop things from happening in their life right now. They prefer not to be participating in them, so this inflammation develops as an outbreak. The outbreak is a response to the discomfort they are experiencing within.

These people are in a position maybe for the first time in their life where they are being forced to prove themselves, or their inadequacy as they see it. Earlier in life they had more control over what was seen of their capabilities. Now, as they are getting older they cannot control what will show through in their ability.

These people have spent their whole lives believing that they were not good enough - *not questioning* it, but rather *believing* it. Their pride they hold high, so anything that would prove to diminish this, they have in the past avoided. They intentionally have avoided many things in their life that they could not control. Now, they are not able to avoid these things that they cannot control from being displayed about their self like they use to. They are getting older and it does show through that they are not as capable *as they used to be*. This is the key. What they often do in attempts to have this not show through is to *not do* anything. In their mind, then this inadequacy will never have to show through. They want what they think about themselves to never be seen. This is their biggest fear.

Their soul learning is to get past their pride and realize that they may not be able to do all things, or even what they used to do, but this is not an indication of how adequate they are. Adequacy is an internal measurement, not external. As long as one tries to prove this externally they will engage in this battle forever and remain ill. They need to come to see that they are good enough just as they are. They don't have to hide their inabilities; we all lack ability in certain things. This is part of being human.

S

SCALP DISORDERS

All scalp dis-eases transpire due to a lack of faith in oneself. These individuals lack self-confidence. They are facing a crisis at this time in their life where the picture around them is reflecting to them a grim scene. Life is not pleasant for them at this time, so it provokes a reflection to them of uncertainty about *who they are and what they may become*. Their *ideal self* doesn't match their *actual self*. Who they would

106

like to be and what they would like to have accomplished in their life, their status, is not what they desire. This is rather troubling for them to deal with.

These individuals should not use external standards and expectations when judging who they are and what they can become. They judge themselves so harshly that it almost seems useless to continue to try. This provokes them to give up internally and therefore close down their energy and stop trying. When they stop trying, they stop the life force from feeding them to continue to thrive in the game of life. There inability to be receptive to life's energies is reduced therefore stimulation to the head and scalp is blocked. This leads to scalp disorders.

These individuals' soul learning is to realize that they cannot *blame* themselves for what life has brought them so far, and thus give up. Rather, they need to *take charge* of their situations and do something about changing the future. They need to leave the past behind and now focus on the future.

The soul learning for these individuals is to stop trying to avoid what is bothering them and learn to confront the situation and express their feelings to the person(s) involved.

SCIATIC NERVE
(SEE ALSO BACK PROBLEMS)

These people put an overabundant amount of stress upon themselves to *perform*, like all other back-related problems. Once the nerve gets involved with a back problem this indicates that not only is one putting an excessive amount of energy into succeeding, but they are also judging this success based on their own personal *integrity*.

These individuals *question themselves*. They question whether they are good enough right down to their very structure, their bones. They don't have strong hopes for themselves. They usually have a self-confidence that is low because others have battered them. They feel that they don't get support from others, so they often do a lot of things on their own to *prove themselves*. They run themselves down by doing so many things externally and are unable to find self-worth internally to keep holding themselves up.

These individuals need to see the worth in themselves so that they can hold themselves up strong internally, and then it will show externally. Their soul learning is to overcome their fear of *personal failure*. They need to see themselves as a **winner** first, before they do anything, not after, and then judging it based on whether or not they were good enough.

SCOLIOSIS

Individuals who acquire this dis-ease have an inability to *stand up for themselves.* Their posture is how they represent themselves to the world. They stand back in the crowd, not to be noticed. These people don't make a place for themselves in life. They take whatever is handed to them. This action of theirs cannot carry on; they need to let themselves be known.

Their soul learning is to take a stand for *who they are* by expressing who they are: their thoughts, feelings and beliefs. This is how they can make themselves known, instead of standing back and not allowing themselves to be heard.

By having such a dis-ease they have to learn how to stand straight, through exercise, braces, chiropractic, surgery, etc. All of these actions that they do externally in their life to deal with this dis-ease are equally going on internally, all of which will teach them to **stand up for themselves**.

SHINGLES – HERPES ZOSTER

The shingles virus is one that activates on command of certain emotional strife. When emotional strife reaches a peak point in the individual's life, shingles are sure to rise. What commonly brings about this activation is one having suffered much grief over another individual in their life. Somebody in their life is triggering an emotional upset that really gets under their skin. Because this bothers them so much within, it eats away at them and thus induces a reaction that results in an outbreak in the form of shingles.

The emotion involved is fear of self-placement. The individual that is bothering them is causing them fear over their position in life. What it boils down to is that the individual threatens their emotional (not physical) position of receiving *love.* If there is any threat of this nature later in their life, then this virus is capable to rise again.

When feeling this emotional strife, they feel as if someone is taking them over. They almost feel smothered. So in response, instead of coming out, they go within, closing them self off. Therefore, the way this emotional fear and anger comes out or releases is through the skin.

Having this virus that releases itself through the skin is a way of letting the individual with this virus let off some steam. Yet truly the individual needs to be expressing these emotions by letting them come out in other ways, rather than just through the skin as a last resort. Their soul learning is to learn how to *confront* the individual who is bothering them by expressing their feelings that are upsetting them.

SHOULDER PROBLEMS

Those that have a common occurrence of pressure on their shoulders are putting a enormous amount of pressure upon themselves. The phrase *"carrying the weight of the world on their shoulders"* is a perfect fit for them. They are always running, going and doing, trying to take care of everything – and trying to take care of things that they are not even capable of taking care of. They run themselves down a lot doing this. These people have put very high expectations upon themselves. Things run in an *orderly fashion* for them. This is their motto that they like to live by. In fact, their life is often too organized. They are too fact-oriented, allowing little room for possibilities, new ideas or ways of doing things in their life. The more that they put this pressure on themselves to run in this orderly fashion, the more the pressure they will put on their shoulders. This pressure is induced by them self because they are trying to force things to go the way they wish them to be. They get very caught up in doing what it is that they *want*, rather than what needs to be. They don't want to look at what must be. They are too busy spending time trying to change the way things are.

Their soul learning is to learn to look at what their soul is guiding them to do, being open to possibilities. This requires them to learn to be open to different possibilities about the situation they're trying to face and force. They need to look for a new way to go about it. They are forcing something, and nature is telling them that there is an alternative way that they need to approach this situation that they are being resistant to. They need to *be open.*

SINUS HEADACHES

Sinus headaches are similar to, yet different from normal headaches in the way that the mental energy is more precisely located with the sinuses. This relates to something that is right under the individual's nose that they are having a hard time understanding.

As they look at this situation that is bothering them they ask, *"Can I, or will it ever happen?"* To them, based on their facts, the hope looks dim, although they continue to keep searching for answers. They are too caught up in figuring out how to make it work; yet they lack both all the facts and the possibilities to make a clear analysis or decision. Their soul learning is to open up and look at what's right in front of them in their life in a new and different way, searching for options they were closed-minded to before.

SKIN PROBLEMS

In all cases of skin problems, one is *annoyed* or *bothered* by someone or about something. Someone or something has gotten under their skin, and they can't just let it go. Although they have tried to conceal it, they ultimately cannot avoid it. They have tried to close themselves off from it as a way of coping with it, yet what is irritating them inside must find a way to release, and in this case it is coming out through the skin. As it comes out, it can be seen as a reminder to them letting them know that they must now deal with this situation by confronting it, by expressing their thoughts, feelings and beliefs about it, in the best manner they can. It cannot just be left alone. It is eating away at them.

Someone or something that they are letting get to them bothers anybody who has a skin irritation, in any manner. They have a certain perspective that they are not willing to budge on about a specific situation. Overall, they are being closed-minded about it, not wanting to see any other possibilities about it. They have a one-track mind.

Their soul learning is that they need to open themselves up to look at things differently in their life from different perspectives or points of view. They can then let go of the situation that is bothering them once it is understood, but to understand it, they need to look at it and approach it in a different way. Only by being open to new possibilities about the circumstance or situation can they come to terms with what is bothering them and be able to put it to rest. Therefore, they will no longer be irritated and their skin problems will begin to alleviate.

SPASMS

Spasms are a reaction of the muscles to a high level of stress in the body. The body internally is having a difficult time dealing with a sudden overload of stress in one's life.

These individuals are in a state of *fear*. The spasms are a reaction to the fear they are encountering within, just as when we experience fear on the outside. When we get scared by something, "What do we do?" Jump! This is similar to what occurs within.

The individual is suffering from some insecurity. They are going through a process in which the path has a hazy light on it and the details look dim. They feel too exposed and open to anything. They feel they are unable to predict their next step. They don't know what could be coming their way. Everything is all only speculation. There are too many unknown factors. This level of uncertainty is very pain staking for them. They feel very discontented and cannot seem to become pacified, so the body lives on edge with a high level of energy that induces these responses of spasms as a reaction to the fear for a release.

Their soul learning is to learn to relax and feel safe with life. They need to learn to not fear the outcome of things, *knowing* that all things are divine and happen for a reason. There is no need to fear the outcome; our soul has the best interest in mind for the whole of our being, always.

SPINE PROBLEMS
(SEE ALSO BACK PROBLEMS AND/OR DISC PROBLEMS)

When one has problems with their spine, whether minor or major, it indicates that the individual is not allowing things to run smoothly in their life. Along the spine is where all of the energy in our body constantly runs, bringing information to and from the brain and the body. When an individual stops the energy flow for reasons such as uncertainty about life circumstances, they end up affecting the spine itself. The degree of spinal problems is relevant to the degree of blocked energy that one is stopping from freely flowing in their life.

Understand that the reason a person stops the flow of energy in their body is because they are trying to slow things down from happening due to some uncertainty within their life. They are caught up in trying to keep things as they are because they are comfortable, rather than letting them freely become what they need to be. By doing this they end up blocking avenues of opportunities from happening within their life.

These individual's soul learning is that although it makes them feel uneasy and uncertain to just let things happen, they need to remove their control. This is truly the better way. What they may not realize is that by trying to stop things that they feel uncomfortable with in life from happening, they as well stop other things from happening, not just necessarily what they intended. So, overall not only are they stopping what they fear, they are also stopping what they want to be as well.

SPRAINS

Sprains occur because one has put undue stress or *strain* on the body to overdo. One has caused the body pressure to perform when it was unable to. The individual is in circumstances where they are unable to perform, to come up with an answer or decision, and they are forcing themselves to, or are being forced to perform anyway. Yet, at this time they are lost for an answer or a direction. There seems to be too many possibilities, and they cannot seem to find a clear one.

These individual's soul learning is to quit forcing or being forced in a direction.

They need to take time by themselves and think things through. This will give them better clarity as to what decisions they need to make for themselves. They need to take the time they need to come to their direction and decision instead of being forced or feeling forced to make a decision that they are not yet capable of. Through the process of sprains the individual is allowed time to relax and take a break to let things settle and heal. This is what was needed; yet they wouldn't take time and do it on their own. Now the clarity will come through for their decision through the process of this dis-ease.

STONES

The formation of stones is the body's way to try to deal with the overproduction of a particular organ's function. This occurs over a long period of time. This process occurs because the individual has a lot of energy running through the organ due to the individual not having a clear direction somewhere in their life. This energy builds and gets stuck, causing pain. This pain is a signal that *we are stuck*. It is as if we are running in place and not going anywhere. This is due to the fact that we truly don't know where to go.

These individual's soul learning is to take some time, slow down and take a look at what they may wish to be doing. It is truly important that they are in alignment with what their true desires are. The problem is that they don't know what their desires may be. This is the biggest problem they face. Therefore, these individuals need to take some time and evaluate this. Then pick one course of action and follow through with it to see what comes from it. They need to learn not to follow the usual pattern, which involves getting caught off in many different directions, thereby losing their main goal and focus.

For a more definite understanding of this learning it is important to look at where the stone(s) is located and look to the nature of the organ, it's function, and then metaphorically compare that to our life. Understand that this is the process that they are having trouble with in life. Take for example, kidney stones. The kidney acts as the body's natural filtration system to remove toxins from the body. Toxins occur in the body from an overload of negative energy from negative thoughts and feelings of the individual over not having a direction. Their body literally can no longer filter these negative thoughts and feelings they have any longer, resulting in kidney stones.

STREPTOCOCCAL (STREP THROAT)

Individuals who encounter strep throat are individuals that are on a mission in their life to outdo them self. They are overdoing in expressing themselves, not just in terms of speech expression, but also pure expression of oneself and who they are: thoughts, feelings, beliefs and behaviors. These individuals are trying too hard to do. They are overdoing, to the point where they really can't handle what they are doing currently. They feel inadequate about their ability, having a low sense of self-worth. They feel that they can't be successful at what they are doing, so they are trying to overdo to be successful.

These individuals need to realize that they can conquer anything that passes their path in life. God does not give us more than we are able to handle. They need to realize that they are successful at whatever it is that they do. They don't need to do or be more to prove to them self that they are successful. They have already achieved success. Their soul learning is that they need to come to see themselves as already successful at whatever they are doing. Then they can let go of the inner battle to further succeed, thereby no longer overstraining themselves. As they refrain from over expressing themselves, the pain in their throat will lessen and the bacteria will subside.

STROKE

Those who suffer from a stroke have a poise or character about them that holds strong for their beliefs. It's not just a particular belief in something that they are choosing to stand strong for, rather; they hold a strong position on everything. They are *right* and nobody is going to prove them, or show them differently. They are very opinionated people, to the point that they will stand for their opinions even if they take them to the grave with them. These people have a set way of life that they have lived thus far and they are not going to change for no one or nothing. They are being too closed-minded. Their soul learning is to learn to be open-minded, to be open to new ideas and possibilities about all things in life, instead of being closed-minded to others' opinions in life.

They often need to ask themselves, "Is it really worth killing yourself over?" "*Do you always have to be right?*" These two questions are very tough for them because they know life no other way, and really don't see the extreme that they are.

Having a stroke can often help this personality character to change itself. This dis-ease will teach them to become open to other possibilities in life other than their own. Through this process they will not be able to be as tense because they are in fear of another stroke, which will happen until they can learn to relax. This stroke will slow down their capabilities. This is a repercussion for being too closed-mined and *tense*. The more they are tense, the more a stroke is apt to occur.

SWELLING

Swelling occurs when there is an excessive amount of energy that increases in one place too quickly for the body to filter, so it swells. This is induced because of something that has just recently taken place in one's life that they are unable to understand, and they do not know how to deal with it. Because they don't know what else to do to deal with it, the energy turns into fluid over time and builds because it doesn't have a outlet or placement.

When we eat, we secrete our waste through bowel movements. Everything that we have seen, heard, smelled, or experienced subconsciously or consciously, goes in to keep our bodies balanced. There needs to be an equal amount of energy in and an equal amount of energy out. Therefore, when we see, hear and smell different things and do not express it, it stays stuck within. If they don't get expressed, those thoughts and feelings stay inside, thus inducing swelling from the energy backing up.

To understand this issue more fully, it is best to look where the swelling has occurred. A few examples: If the swelling is in the feet, then this represents that one is having trouble taking a certain step in their life. They have become hesitant, and therefore the energy has stopped freely flowing, resulting in a buildup of energy, in this case causing swelling in the feet. If the swelling is of the hands, then it is concerning something that one has just engaged in and they fear its outcome. If the swelling is of the eye then this is concerning something that they just saw that they were unable to understand or deal with.

The soul learning is that they need to learn that even if they didn't know how to deal with the occurrence, that the only way to place the occurrence and deal with it is by going through it, no matter what the results are the overall intention is positive. It helps promote soul growth. By acting it will provoke the energy in the body wherever it may be built up, allowing it to flow freely. If not, and one stays stuck with what to do, the energy will remain built up and the swelling will continue.

T

TEETH PROBLEMS

Individuals who face any problems with their teeth are facing problems with themselves, the way they look, appear, or carry them self through life. Their stature is not satisfactory for them, so it is hidden deep within them. They deny and hide their true feelings, keeping them in to fester. Because they are unhappy with their stature they don't feel significant. Therefore, they don't feel that they have a right to speak up for themselves, to express their thoughts, feelings, and beliefs. They are feeling deep within like they really don't count. Yet, it has gotten to a point where they are coming out. There are situations in their life that are giving them the opportunity to let it out, but they try to *cover it up*. The mouth is the last place left that it can hide before it is to be expressed, so this is the last place they try to store it or stop it. Yet, we can't hide our self and our true feelings too long; eventually they will show through.

Every tooth has a nerve that sends a specific message to the brain every time it is stimulated by eating, drinking, etc. Each tooth has a specific signal, a specific emotional stimulus to deliver. The way one deals with their emotions determines the shape and structure of the teeth, for example, crooked-teeth, under-bites, over bites, etc.

In all cases of teeth problems the individual is having a difficult time with themselves expressing their needs and feelings. These people tend to avoid the way they feel, often trying to forget about their feelings, and eventually just denying them. They don't allow themselves to get the care they need, not just physically, but more importantly here emotionally forgetting about their needs. If there isn't a balance with an equal amount of energy going in and coming out, there will be a problem. This is because they are too busy meeting everybody else's needs and neglecting to speak up for their own needs.

These individual's soul learning is to learn to speak up for their thoughts, feelings and beliefs, realizing that they have a right just as everybody else, regardless of stature. They must learn to speak up even if it requires that they expressing theirs may upset someone else's feelings. Remember that we all need to express ourselves, who we are. If we hold our true self back, we will get sick. Also realize that the individual to whom they need to express their thoughts, feelings and beliefs to, is not there by accident either, so it actually is necessary for both of the souls. These individuals need to stop worrying about everybody else's needs and start concentrating on fulfilling their own needs.

TOOTHACHES:

Simple toothaches come and go, often leading to no particular or greater tooth problems. We acquire toothaches because we are questioning our status or situation in life. The pain is the key or wake-up signal to pay attention: *"What are you trying to hide or avoid from expressing?"* One needs to take a look at their life and clear things up. Don't leave any skeletons in the closet. Their soul learning is to "Speak up what you feel, think and believe."

CAVITIES:

Cavities signifies emotions being buried, cavities state that one has successfully try to decompose something unpleasant that they didn't want to say. Kind of like a kid who eats the candy wrapper so that there was no proof of eating the candy. This is the way the self expels it. Their soul learning is"Don't hide your truth. "

CRACKED TEETH:

Those who have cracked teeth you could say have not been truthful about something that they have kept hidden and have tried to make up for it, yet now it is eating them away. In other words, for them to just decompose it they have to suffer from its effects of the *not truth*. Their soul learning is to "Speak your truths always, at all costs. "

ROOT CANALS:

This concealed emotion has done damage from keeping it in so long. It is displaying itself now because there is a desperate attempt to bring it to the surface. The nerve has reached its maximum point of concealment. This particular emotion has reached its potential. There is an inner suffering left by the person because that tooth no longer has a nerve, or the means to express this particular emotion. Their soul learning is to "Quit grinning and bearing it (grinding your teeth) and speak your truths no matter what the results may be. "

THROAT INFECTION

A general infection of the throat is related to one who has a lot of stored thoughts and feelings about other people and or things that are bothering them and they are not expressing them, particularly to whom they need to.

An infection arises due to one having bothered emotions built up over time with no resolution to put them to rest. So, they will need to go through more experiences to keep reminding them of these thoughts and feelings that they are bothered about, until ultimately so that they can bring resolution to them.

The throat and mouth is one of the last places left for it to stay stored, without truths coming out. In other words, it's right there and they are not saying or expressing what they are truly thinking and feeling about the situation(s) that has them so inflamed.

This soul learning is in relation to them self getting a chance to express all of who they truly are. They need to be who they are instead of thinking and feeling that they don't have the right. They have just as much right to say what they think and feel as the next person. Nothing in life should ever hold them back from being and expressing who they are, their truths.

TUBERCULOSIS

People who contract this dis-ease are those who have become lost in life. They are allowing themselves to fall through the cracks in life. They feel insignificant, so they approach life with the same manner in which they feel about themselves. They *feel* insignificant, so they will act in an insignificant manner. Those suffering from tuberculosis do not center love within, finding a way to love themselves, so therefore they are not out to give love, which translates to not getting involved in life.

Their soul learning is to learn that only getting involved in life can help them come to realize just how significant they really are. This process of engaging in life will help them see that they are just as significant as any other being, allowing them to learn how to love themselves for who they are. Individuals who have acquired such a dis-ease are, crying out to have love, so that they can then feel love for themselves and thus feel good enough about themselves.

U

ULCERS

Individuals who acquire ulcers either peptic or duodenal ulcers, result from the individuals' negative perception of themselves. On the outside they are on top of things. They put up a good front on the outside, yet inside shows the real picture of what they think and believe of themselves.

They are not what they wish to be. They have a conflict between who they are and what they want to be. Rather than accepting themselves for who they are, which is what they need to do, they spend time trying to be more than who they are. By spending so much time trying to be who they are not, what ends up happening is they lose themselves and begin to wonder, *"What am I?" and "Am I me?"*

They are overly sensitive people who are very nitpicky towards themselves and others. The reason they are nitpicky or critical of others is because they are that way with themselves. They are too harsh with themselves. Their soul learning is to lay off themselves and accept themselves for who they are and what they are. They don't have to be better, by trying to be this is what is making them miserable.

UNDERWEIGHT

Individuals who are underweight don't sit around long enough for anything to grow on them. This is the problem in their life in general. They are always the ones busy overdoing things, over-expressing themselves and their opinions.

They are always taking charge of things in life, even things they don't really have charge of yet. This makes them feel like they have things in control in their life. They always have to be over-prepared. The underlying problem is that they have this inner issue where they want to remain in control of how things go, rather than freely being open to what life has to bring their way on even the journey of the day and learning that they may have to change or cancel *plans.*

They keep themselves so busy with so many things, expressing their selves externally that they save very little time to deal with what they need to, which are some inner needs. This is not a good way to avoid them. By not dealing with them they are not able to grow and literally are not even able to put on weight. They are also allowing many other avenues in their life to pass them by.

Their soul learning is to slow down the pace and stop overdoing, forcing, etc. They're holding on to the reins too tight, trying to control everything. They need to allow themselves to be more free-spirited, having faith and realizing everything is divine and learn that the only thing we need to have control over is our own life. They need to deal with what life sends their way, letting things come freely into their life. Accepting this will help them gain and maintain weight.

URINARY INFECTION

One who acquires a urinary infection has some stored and festered feelings that they are not or have not been happy about for a long time. They have been unhappy with the way things have been going and are still going in a particular area in their life. They feel they have no control over it and they are *pissed off* about it. Things aren't going as they should be according to them and there is nothing they can do about it, or won't. It's gotten to the point that they don't even want to look at it any longer.

Their soul learning is that they must take a good look at it and no longer avoid it. Rather they need to face these things in their life that they do not see as appropriate and do something about them, rather than letting them continue on, and doing nothing about them.

V

VARICOSE VEINS

Individual's who have varicose veins, whether severe or minor, are often women who face difficulty with self in accepting their age, because they feel that their capabilities are decreasing, as they are getting older. Varicose veins are also known to come about with an excessive amount of weight: again here the individual is trying to carry more than they are capable of. Varicose veins signify one who is feeling not capable enough to participate in life. They are unsure how to approach life due to the changes in their body. Because of this apprehension the pathway of energy – blood - in the body blocks up and bulges out.

These individuals are having a hard time channeling their energy in life. So, they often sit back and hold back. Yet, the reason that they're holding back is because they are afraid to try and prove themselves. *"What if they fail? "* They are in fear of failure, so they don't want to be in the spotlight in case they fail.

These individual's soul learning is to find a safe environment, which includes support from family and friends, to allow them space to do what they may wish without any expectation on them. They need to learn to handle their own expectations before they will be able to handle the expectations placed on them from others. They need to prove to themselves first in their own safe and quiet way.

VENEREAL (SEXUALLY TRANSMITTED) DIS-EASES

Those who acquire any venereal or sexually transmitted dis-eases' have got themselves in over their head with some of the decisions that they have made. They are apprehensive about being their true self. They don't want to face this: They are busy being stuck on where they want to be more than where they are. They are having trouble taking the steps they need to get where they want to get, because they don't feel able or capable to get there. They need to face who they are and where they are truly at in life. They need to stop trying to be more than they are. This is what got them into their problem in the first place.

These individuals hesitate to make decisions because they feel they are not able, that they don't have the ability to make the appropriate or right decisions. This is the case because they see little hope and few possibilities, because they are not being open-minded enough to look at different ways, ideas and possibilities to make not only small decisions in life, but also bigger decisions regarding their life overall, about where they are going and what they need to be doing in life.

Because of their inability to make the right decisions in their eyes, they hold back and often don't make decisions, which makes them look *irresponsible* or like they're making inappropriate decisions, which only perpetuates the same cycle.

Overall, they are not content with their life. They don't see the possibilities of where life is going for them. They feel overlooked, as if they aren't special. They need to learn that they can stand out in a crowd by just being who they are. Their soul learning is that they must face, accept, and love themselves for who they are. Then they can work on going and getting where they want to be in life.

We all have a unique and important purpose on this earth different from all others, but none the less important. It is important that we be who we are: make decisions based on the knowledge we do have. By not making decisions the progression of life halts. Not doing this due to fear is only holding us, and our life back from going forward.

W

WARTS

Those who acquire warts are those that have a nature about them that cannot just let things be as they are, or happen as they do. They are considered *"worry warts."* That's not to say that anyone who worries will have warts, or that warts are the only thing caused by worrying. This is not true. Rather, it is worrying in a particular manner that will cause warts.

These individuals have to have their hands in everything in life. They have a hard time just accepting life and situations in life as they are. They want things to be as they wish, to the point where they try to put extensive effort into changing things. Although they often cannot do anything about it, to them they feel like they are doing. To them it's something that they must do. These individuals bring about worrying because they are always trying to remain in control.

Their soul learning is to learn that things cannot always be as they wish in their life. Ultimately, what needs to be will be for their soul learning. But it is much easier if we don't fight the divine plan, stop worrying, and know that all things are divine. Then they will be able to accept things in their life as they are.

WEIGHT GAIN

The mystery of why one gains weight is a big question in our society. The reason that one would begin to gain weight is because of a backup of emotional energy that is not freely released from the individual. They are having a hard time with something that they cannot freely accept or let go of, so they keep that emotional pain in, not expressing their feelings about it. This excessive energy within the body is reflected throughout the body. This emotional stuffing, so to speak, that is held within the body soon shows outside.

When an individual starts to gain weight they become sluggish. They start to slow down their pace of life and give up a little; thus they start to push life and opportunities away from them. This occurs to begin with because the individual experienced some type of emotional insecurity that has left them questioning whether they are *good enough*. They don't feel that they can live up to the standards in life, so what they do instead is do nothing. If they don't put them self out there, then they won't have to face the possible feeling of *rejection*.

Their soul learning is that the only way they can overcome this feeling of rejection is by facing it, by putting them self back out there in life and realizing that they are *good enough* just the way they are. Eventually, the more they do this the easier it will be to express their feelings, who they are. By expressing their feelings, they will be able to freely accept and thus let go of this emotional pain, excess energy and finally weight.

INDEX

ABDOMINAL CRAMPING 25

ABSCESSES...26

ACIDIC STOMACH 27

ACNE 27

ATTENTION DEFICIT DISORDER 28

ACQUIRED IMMUNODEFICIENCY SYNDROME....................30

ALCOHOLISM 31

ALLERGIES..32

ALZHEIMER'S DIS-EASE 33

ANEMIA..34

ANOREXIA 34

ANXIETY 35

ARTERIOSCLEROSIS 36

ARTHRITIS – OSTEOARTHRITIS 36

ASTHMA...37

ATHEROSCLEROSIS 38

ATHLETES FEET 38

BACK PROBLEMS(Lower. Middle and Upper Back) 39

Lower Back..39

Middle Back 40

Upper Back 40

BALDNESS...40

BLADDER PROBLEMS..41

BLEEDING(In general) 41

BLOOD CLOTS 42

BLOOD PRESSUREHigh and Low......................................43

BREAST LUMPS..44

BROKEN BONES 44

BRONCHITIS..45

BRUISE...45

BUNIONS...46

BURSITIS..46

CANCER...47

CANDIDASIS...48

CARPAL TUNNEL SYNDROME...48

CATARACTS..49

CELLULITE..50

CEREBRAL PALSY..50

CHEST COLDS(See also Congestion)..................................51

CIRCULATION...51

COLIC..52

COLON..52

COLITIS...52

COMA..53

CONGESTION(See also Chest Colds).................................54

CONJUCTIVITIES..54

CONSTIPATION...55

CONVULSIONS..55

COUGHS...56

CROHN'S DISEASE...56

DEPRESSION..57

DIABETES...57

DIARRHEA...58

DISC PROBLEMS(See Back Problems)...............................58

DIGESTIVE PROBLEMS..58

DRUG ADDICTION..59

EARACHES...60

EDEMA...60

EMPHYSEMA...61

ENDOMETRIOSIS...61

EPILESPSY..63

EPSTEIN BARR VIRUS..63

EYES – FARSIGHTED..64

EYES – NEARSIGHTED...65

FATIGUE..65

FEARS...66

FEVER...67

FOOD POISIONING...68

GALL BLADDER...68

GLAUCOMA..68

GOUT 69

GUM PROBLEMS 70

HEAD COLDS(See also Colds)..70

HEADACHES...71

HEARING PROBLEMS..71

HEART ATTACK 72

HEARTBURN 72

HEMORRHOIDS..73

HEPATITIS 73

HERNIA..74

HIVES...74

HODGKINS DIS-EASE..75

HUNTINGTON'S DIS-EASE 75

HYPERTHYRODISM 76

HYPOGLYCEMIA..77

HYPOTHYROIDISM..77

HYSTERIA 77

IMPOTENCE...78

INFECTION (Bacterial)(See also Infection - Viral) 78

INFECTION (Viral)(See also Infection - Bacterial)....................79

INFERTILITY..80

INFLAMATION (ACUTE) 81

INFLUENZA(See also Infections – Viral) 81

INSOMNIA..82

ITCHING...82

JAUNDICE 83

JOINT INFLAMMATION 83

KIDNEY PROBLEMS 84

KNEE PROBLEMS(General) 84

LIVER 85

LOU GEHRIG'S DIS-EASE 86

LOW IMMUNE SYSTEM 87

LUNG PROBLEMS 88

LYMPHATIC PROBLEMS(Glands and nodes)...........................88

MENENGITIS 89
MENOPAUSAL PROBLEMS 89
MIGRAINE HEADACHES 90
MONONUCLEOSIS 91
MOUTH SORES – CANKER SORES 91
MULTIPLE SCLEROSIS 92
MUSCULAR DYSTROPHY 92
NAUSEA 93
NECK 93
NERVE PROBLEMS 94
NEURALGIA 95
NEURITIS 96
OBESITY 96
OSTEOPOROSIS 97
PANIC DISORDER 98
PARALYSIS 100
PARASITES 100
PARKINSON'S DISEASE 101
PNEUMONIA 102
POLIOMYELITIS 102
PREMENSTRUAL SYNDROME 103
PROSTATE PROBLEMS 103
PSORIASIS 104
RASH 105
RHEUMATOID ARTHRITIS 106
SCALP DISORDERS 106
SCIATIC NERVE(See also Back Problems) 107
SCOLIOSIS 108
SHINGLES – HERPES ZOSTER 108
SHOULDER PROBLEMS 109
SINUS HEADACHES 109
SKIN PROBLEMS 110
SPASMS 110
SPINE PROBLEMS(See also Back Problems and/or Disc Problems) 111
SPRAINS 111
STONES 112
STREPTOCOCCAL (Strep Throat) 112

STROKE..113

SWELLING...114

TEETH PROBLEMS..114

TOOTHACHES:...115

CAVITIES:...116

CRACKED TEETH:...116

ROOT CANALS:..116

THROAT INFECTION..116

TUBERCULOSIS...117

ULCERS...117

UNDERWEIGHT...118

URINARY INFECTION...118

VARICOSE VEINS..119

VENEREAL (SEXUALLY TRANSMITTED) DIS-EASES...................119

WARTS..120

WEIGHT GAIN...120

ISBN 141206544-5